"A thoughtful volume filled wit[...] emotional eaters everywhere."

—Madelyn H. Fernstrom, [...], [...], director of UPMC Weight Management Center, professor at the University of Pittsburgh Medical Center

"Albers's soup-to-nuts list of creative, accessible, self-soothing tips will undoubtedly help anyone who has struggled with dieting, food, or body image. Beyond that, her exercises in mindfulness, deep breathing, and journaling are top-notch tools for finding balance in life overall."

—Leslie Goldman, author of *Locker Room Diaries*

"Albers has done it again! *50 Ways to Soothe Yourself Without Food* makes complex psychological concepts simple and accessible. I highly recommend you buy this book if you have ever turned to food for comfort and want to learn a new way of coping."

—Kathleen Burns Kingsbury, LMHC, CPCC, coauthor of *Weight Wisdom* and founder of KBK Connections, Inc.

"You don't have to be worried about your waistline to reap life-changing benefits from Albers's easy-to-follow guidance. Reading this little book will boost your mood, reduce stress, and provide soothing alternatives to that next dessert! I highly recommend it."

—Amy Weintraub, author of *Yoga for Depression* and director of the LifeForce Yoga Healing Institute

50 ways to soothe yourself without food

SUSAN ALBERS, PSY.D.

New Harbinger Publications, Inc.

Distributed in Canada by Raincoast Books

Copyright © 2009 by Susan Albers
New Harbinger Publications, Inc.
5674 Shattuck Avenue
Oakland, CA 94609
www.newharbinger.com

Cover design by Amy Shoup; Cover illustration by Sara Christian;
Text design by Amy Shoup and Michele Waters-Kermes;
Acquired by Catharine Sutker; Edited by Kayla Sussell

Library of Congress Cataloging-in-Publication Data

Albers, Susan, Psy.D.
  50 ways to soothe yourself without food / Susan Albers.
      p. cm.
  Includes bibliographical references.
  ISBN-13: 978-1-57224-676-8 (pbk. : alk. paper)
  ISBN-10: 1-57224-676-6 (pbk. : alk. paper) 1. Compulsive eating. 2. Food habits--Psychological aspects. 3. Meditation--Therapeutic use. I. Title. II. Title: Fifty ways to soothe yourself without food.
  RC552.C65A43 2009
  616.85'26--dc22

                              2009023473

14   13   12

10   9   8   7

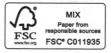

To Brookie,
May you be blessed with patience and fortitude.

Contents

acknowledgments

As always, I must thank my clients, readers of the Eating Mindfully series, and friends who generously shared their strategies and tips for soothing themselves without food. Their stories always inspire me to keep working on finding ways to help ease the suffering caused by eating problems. It is my sincere hope that you will gain some useful strategies for comforting and nurturing yourself from reading this book.

My gratitude to the people who soothe me best: John Bowling, Brooklyn Bowling, Dr. Victoria Gould, Jane Lindquist Lesniewski, Betsy Beyer Swope, Dr. Jason Greif, Eric Lingenfelter, Dr. Angela Albers, Linda Serotta, Carmela and Dr. Thomas Albers, and John, Rhonda, and Jim Bowling.

This book would not be possible without the editors and staff at New Harbinger Publications. A special thank you to Catharine Sutker and Kayla Sussell.

introduction

On days like today, I could eat everything that isn't nailed down. I find myself sneaking into the kitchen after getting both kids to bed. I rummage through the refrigerator for something to eat. I justify my nibbling by telling myself that after such a hard day, I deserve something satisfying. Munching makes me feel good. It's instant bliss. I forget about all my chores and stress. And after all the leftovers are gone, I still feel like I need something else. So I open up a box of cookies. I can't stop eating them until I am way passed stuffed. Why does eating feel so good in the moment, and then I feel so much worse than when I started? —Rachel

Does this sound familiar? When Rachel needs comfort, she needs it now! A nagging boss, demanding kids, and never-ending housework all seem to vanish for a moment—just as long as she is eating. Munching on potato chips provides a seductive moment of calming and soothing. But just a few minutes after she swallows the last morsel, the soothing effect vanishes and she is filled with regret and guilt. Rachel's relationship with food sums up the way most emotional eaters feel, sometimes on a daily basis. Eating has an amazingly contradictory power. It can relax and calm your nerves, while at the same time, it can drive you crazy.

When you eat to soothe yourself, it is generally what most of us call stress eating or emotional eating. These terms describe the times you eat specifically to calm down, numb out, or elevate, prolong, lessen, or avoid your feelings. Notice, however, that emotional eating and stress eating are different. *Stress eating* means consuming food in response to feeling overwhelmed or upset. *Emotional eating* includes eating done not to relieve hunger, but in response to any kind of feeling, even pleasant ones like joy and surprise. Yes, it's true. Even good feelings can lead to overeating. Sometimes you eat because it makes you feel good and you don't want that feeling to stop. In Rachel's case, just about any kind of demand on her time prompted her to eat for emotional reasons.

Rachel's emotional eating was becoming a problem. The same cycle was repeating over and over again. Stress. Need comfort. Need to eat. Feel relief. Feel good. Positive feeling fades. Feel guilt. Need soothing. More stress about guilt and weight gain. Begin cycle again. Although eating provided a temporary emotional patch, the major downside was that she was gaining weight. She hated stepping on the scale, because every time she weighed herself the numbers seemed to go up. It didn't matter whether she was experiencing a major or a minor stress. Each time she felt stressed, she went straight to food for a quick pick-me-up. Rachel couldn't understand why she continually sought food for comfort when it caused her so much distress about her weight. It just didn't make sense.

This book explains why people like Rachel—and like you— fall into the trap of eating to soothe yourselves. It covers some of the reasons that make emotional eating so seductive and comforting. As you read, you'll be taking a closer look at your emotional eating for the purpose of conquering it. You'll also learn some practical solutions.

Essentially, if you eliminate eating as your main source of comfort, you have to find something helpful to put in its place. In this book, there are over fifty tips and techniques for doing just that. The initial techniques and tips are based on the concept of mindfulness, which is a clinically sound way to calm and soothe both your body and your mind. You will also learn mindful coping skills that will help you to better regulate your emotions. To put it simply, *mindfulness* is the state of awareness. When you are truly aware of what you are feeling and approach your feelings with a nonjudgmental attitude, you can find healthy ways to deal with whatever kind of discomfort you might be trying to numb out with food. Say good-bye to comfort foods and hello to using your mind and body to cope with emotional eating.

my background

As you read this book, you'll notice that I refer to the clients I work with in my psychotherapy practice. I am a clinical psychologist who was trained at the University of Denver and completed a postdoctoral fellowship at Stanford University. Over the last ten years, I have focused on treating clients who are struggling with dieting, body image, anorexia, bulimia, and binge-eating disorder. Many of the examples that I use in this book are adapted from my clients' experiences and stories.

the mystery of emotional eating

I am sad, I eat.
I am irritated with my mother, I eat.
I am frustrated with myself, I eat.
I am happy about my new apartment, I eat.
—Melanie

Many eating problems aren't really about food. They are about self-soothing. *Self-soothing techniques* are methods to calm and relax your body and mind, as well as soothe your nerves. They are the actions you take every day to calm yourself down. The absence of self-soothing techniques is why many diet books help people only up to a certain point. Too often, they don't help their readers lose weight in the first place. Then if the weight is lost, they don't tell their readers how to keep it off over the long term. Diet books address only what you eat. They guide you to make nutritional changes. But far too often they don't cover the reason why you consume too much food.

Sometimes it isn't about what you eat during meals. Your weight gain may be due to the extra calories that come from stress or emotional eating. Unfortunately, diet books seldom tell you how to replace food with other comforting and pleasurable substitutes. Nor do they provide practical and realistic examples of how to deal effectively with emotional eating. Without these elements, managing your weight becomes nearly impossible.

Many people have been taught very ineffective ways to self-soothe from an early age. These ways are mainly about finding an escape parachute to avoid whatever is bothering you. The message is distract yourself, focus on things that feel good, or entertain yourself. Typically, self-soothing means turning to food, TV, gambling, alcohol, work, the Internet, or drugs. For a short time, these activities can take the edge off feeling stressed. In the long run, however, they are temporary solutions that actually can become the problem, even an addiction.

Stress eating, which initially may have helped you cope with feeling frazzled, can evolve into the problem of binge eating and become the source of your distress rather than the comfort that eases your distress. Many people have a very low tolerance for distress. The moment they begin to feel uncomfortable, they look for anything to get rid of that feeling. Quick! However, what is really needed is a solid way to cope with and endure these uncomfortable feelings.

Every day, people find lots of different ways to soothe themselves. Some are helpful and some are not. Activities like exercising, taking a nap, or calling a friend are healthy behaviors for unwinding after a stressful day. Other ways are not good for you and may damage your health and relationships. In fact, some self-soothing behaviors can even be harmful in the long run, like playing games on the computer for hours or numbing yourself out with alcohol. Some of the many ways that people soothe themselves with food are discussed below.

examples of self-soothing with food

This list will provide you with some indications that you may be using food to work through your feelings. This is not an exhaustive list but only some common examples of behaviors that people engage in when using food to deal with stress:

- Eating puts you into a trancelike state or numbs you out.

- Chewing and munching on something feel good.

- Grazing (eating when you aren't hungry, but you can't stop yourself) numbs you.

- Cravings start up from feeling any emotion, whether positive or negative.

- Searching for something to eat, but not being able to find something satisfying.

- Continuing to eat because you can't determine or find what it is that you want to eat.

- Continuing to eat even when it feels like it will never be enough.

- Experiencing a great sense of relief while you are eating.

- Feeling an intense need for something good tasting inside your mouth.

- Experiencing every emotion as hunger. (This makes it hard to know what you are really feeling.)

- Eating as a way to relax.

- Eating immediately after a stressful event or when you are nervous.

- Making the connection and saying, "I'm only eating this candy bar because I am so stressed-out."

- Eating foods you don't even like because they are there and you need comfort.

- Eating to stave off boredom.

- Feeling emotionally empty most of the time despite being well-fed physically.

- Seeking a particular kind of food like, chocolate, because it seems to change your mood.

- Preparing or buying treats so that you'll have them just in case you'll "need" them.

- Tending to overeat at important or stressful events like family reunions and business meetings.

- Eating leads to guilt when you do it for soothing rather than to stop physical hunger.

who is this book for?

This is a great book for all types of emotional eaters. If you use food to soothe yourself, it is truly worth your time to read through all the chapters and try the techniques. We've all experienced emotional eating at one time or another. Men, women, teens, adults—just about everyone uses food to regulate their emotions to some degree. This includes normal eaters (people who don't have eating issues), as well as dieters and those with eating disorders (Macht 2008; Spoor et al. 2007).

For some people, emotional eating is a minor issue. It is done only on rare occasions and in little ways. Gobbling a chocolate brownie to deal with a particularly bad case of PMS symptoms is a good example. Munching nervously on popcorn during a scary movie is another. Even gorging yourself on ice cream after a stressful day can be an acceptable indulgence. Giving yourself this kind of comfort might not be a big deal in the grand scheme of things. But you want to be very cautious that it doesn't become a habit. Nor do you want eating chocolate to be the only method you turn to for soothing each time you have PMS or a bad day. There are other effective options like taking a hot bath, exercising, or meditating. These methods address the problem of stress more directly and don't make you feel guilty or leave you wanting to beat yourself up later for using them.

For many other people, however, eating to self-soothe is a daily, chronic struggle. They do it so often that they become trapped in a vicious cycle they can't break out of. If you have chronic issues with eating or using food to tranquilize yourself, you might have binge-eating disorder or another eating disorder.

In general, *binge-eating disorder* is characterized by frequent and repeated overeating to alleviate stress or other negative feelings. This disorder may be present when your primary means of coping is to eat, and it is not just something you do now and then. You may feel that eating takes up most of your time and energy. You also may feel that your life revolves around eating to the point that it has become difficult to carry out your daily routine.

If you suspect that you have some of the symptoms of binge-eating disorder (or any other eating disorder), it would be to your benefit to obtain additional support and treatment from a mental health professional and a physician to make sure that you are adequately addressing the issue. Reading this book is a great first step, but it's important to get the right kind of treatment as well.

Picking up this book is a fantastic first move. You have just begun a new chapter in your life. You've begun to explore healthy ways to deal with the stress in your life. Keep in mind that it isn't easy to give up food as a source of comfort. It will take time.

gender issues

Although many of the examples in this book are geared toward women, the tips to be found in it apply to all emotional eaters whether they are male or female. If you are a man who is reading this book, you can extrapolate from the examples and tailor the techniques to fit your lifestyle. For example, if you don't enjoy gardening, perhaps you might notice that fishing provides similar benefits to those listed under this technique—it gets you outside and puts you in a relaxed state.

It is also important to point out that this book has many examples and quotes from people coping with overeating problems. However, undereating and restrictive eating habits are also linked to deficits in self-soothing. So if you use restrictive eating to calm yourself or to feel in control of your emotions, consider using these healthy coping mechanisms instead.

five helpful ways to soothe yourself

The fifty soothing techniques in this book are grouped into five major skill areas: mindfulness techniques, strategies to change your thoughts, strategies to calm your body, finding distractions, and gaining support. After you learn about the concept of self-soothing in this introduction and chapter 1, you will learn how to get started in chapter 2. Then you will read about the basic principles of mindfulness in chapter 3. Here is a brief description of what this book holds in store for you.

Mindfulness Meditation Techniques

Mindfulness is defined as being keenly aware of what you are feeling and thinking in the moment, in an open and accepting way. It is both an experience and an attitude. The concept is over twenty-five hundred years old and is still used in modern therapies and healing practices. Mindfulness techniques are well researched and clinically proven to have healing properties for the mind and body (Baer 2003; Proulx 2008; Shapiro et al. 2008). The techniques teach people how to tolerate distress rather than avoid it.

In chapter 3, you will learn how to adopt a mindful attitude of awareness. Modern life is so busy that many people go through their days zoned out, unaware of many of the feelings that lead them to eat for emotional reasons. When you are mindful, you tune in to your mind and body. You can calm your emotions through compassionate inner self-talk, meditation, and breathing exercises.

Mindfulness skills provide a realistic approach because you often can't get rid of the person or event that's causing you stress, such as an untidy spouse or a difficult job assignment. Instead, you have to learn to cope with the people and events that will continue to be a part of your everyday life, even though they tend to drive you crazy. Mindfulness is a perfect choice for self-soothing because it's an easy, straightforward alternative to eating.

Change Your Thoughts, Change Your Eating

In chapter 4 you will learn new ways to think. The more aware you are of the way you think, the better able you are to prevent negative thoughts from triggering stress eating. Mindful thinking, affirmations, guided imagery, and realistic statements are all techniques that help to interrupt the flow of upsetting thoughts that are at the root of stress eating. Positive thinking and optimistic self-talk can help you alter self-defeating thoughts that serve only to exacerbate stress eating.

Soothing Sensations to Calm and Relax Your Body

When you are mindful of your body, you get to know how your body reacts to stress and emotions. In chapter 5, you'll learn how to relax in a natural way without the aid of food. You can use your body as a tool for healing by doing self-massage, exercise, relaxation techniques, and yoga.

Mindful Distraction

Distraction is helpful when you engage in a behavior that is incompatible with eating. In chapter 6, you'll think about activities that can keep you occupied, entertained, and away from the kitchen. These distractions can lift your mood, engage your attention, and be stimulating enough to lessen your urge to eat. Mindful distraction is not done to avoid your feelings but to interrupt unproductive brooding and negative habits.

Soothing Support

One of the best ways to avoid falling into the trap of mindless eating is to find helpful social support. There is nothing more soothing than some comforting words from a friend or connecting with the world in a new way. However, finding such social support can be a challenge. Chapter 7 will give you some concrete ideas on how to reach out to others instead of to your refrigerator for comfort and support.

practice is your best life preserver

It's very important to practice using the self-soothing techniques in this book before you need them. You can't expect to put them into practice in the middle of a very strong urge to eat unless you've done some preliminary practicing. If you wait until you need them, it will be like trying to learn how to swim while you are drowning. You need to be a strong swimmer to deal with a huge wave of emotion. At first, these techniques might take some work or feel uncomfortable. But you want to get so good at doing them that by the time you need to use them, they will seem like second nature.

Coping vs. Blissful

The overarching goal for this book is to help people cope with whatever is driving their urge to emotionally eat. Notice that the goal isn't to erase all of the pain, stress, and frustration complicating your life. Nor is it to obtain pleasure. In other words, don't expect that these exercises will make you feel ecstatic, giddy, or joyous. Those feelings are very different from soothing and calming yourself. If the techniques help you to avoid, reduce, or delay emotional eating, consider this to be a great success.

Eastern philosophies are clear about the notion of suffering. We all suffer. No one can escape it. This is why coping skills are so essential. When you try to escape pain through numbing out or external pick-me-ups, you can unintentionally make the problem worse. If you are an emotional eater, this isn't new news to you. As a result, you may want to really focus on mindful coping. Let this be your main objective.

1 why is eating so soothing?

I love comfort food. My favorite is homemade macaroni and cheese. I'd choose it any day over a gourmet meal. Those little noodles have an amazing ability to make me feel warm and cozy, even when I'm frazzled. I don't understand why eating comfort food makes me feel this good. Maybe it's biological? Or perhaps eating gooey mac and cheese reminds me of being a kid? Why is it like waving a magic wand over my mood? —Kendra

Imagine for a moment two women, Jennifer and Cindy. They both have had a stressful day at work due to their critical and irrational boss. Jennifer begins snacking the moment she gets home, as a way to calm down. Cindy, on the other hand, calls a friend to vent about her terrible day. Why does one woman cope with her irritation by nibbling on snacks while the other turns to a friend to find comfort? You'll find the answer in this chapter, which will cover some theories about how healthy and unhealthy coping mechanisms develop and are maintained. You'll also learn why it is so important to find a nonfood alternative to pacify your mind and body.

theories of self-soothing

Self-soothing is a term coined by the branches of psychology called self psychology and attachment theory. According to these disciplines, the ability to regulate your feelings is at the core of your well-being. *Regulating feelings* simply means that you can temper strong emotions like anger and sadness. You are able to tolerate things that get you really upset and stressed-out without crumbling or falling to pieces. You've probably witnessed people who are very good at self-soothing. They seem able to let things go. Sometimes they look at the bright side of a difficult situation. They cope with stress without turning to methods that could make it worse or be harmful to them. They have the confidence that things will work out, no matter what happens.

You also know people who have no or little ability to self-soothe. When they hit a problem, they fall apart like an eggshell fracturing into hundreds of pieces. They are unable to put the pieces back together. The problem might cause them to become irritable or frazzled. They may have a hard time getting over whatever is bothering them. Sometimes, in extreme cases, people without self-soothing skills can't even function. They have trouble getting up in the morning, going to work, or taking care of themselves.

According to attachment theory, your primary caregivers are the first people to teach you self-soothing skills. As a toddler, when you fall down and scrape your knee, you begin to internalize the caring and calming words your parents say to you while they are picking you up. Your parents also help by rocking you and talking in a slow, soothing voice. One or both parents may also kiss your knee.

As an adult, when you experience a big crisis or an emotional pitfall, you're likely to have a repertoire of calming and soothing words in your memory that you can use to talk yourself through the problem. These calming words became paired with the soothing physiological responses that took place when a parent calmed you down by rocking you. So talking yourself through a crisis tends to automatically trigger the reduction of your physiological reactions associated with stress. You also may find yourself seeking a hug from a loved one. The hug comforts you because you grew up with a parent's touch as a source of support and reassurance.

If you did not learn self-soothing from a parent early on, a hug may not help you at all. Moreover, without early experiences of self-soothing, you may be at a loss for what to say to yourself to work through how you feel. The intensity of your emotion can be so great that you become paralyzed or overwhelmed by how you are feeling. If this is your habitual response to stressful situations, most likely you weren't taught the words you need to soothe yourself. Many people with eating problems have a lot of difficulty putting into words how they feel.

Although your parents may have set the stage for your self-soothing abilities, they weren't the only people who influenced the development of this ability. You may have had other role models in your life who taught you how to self-soothe. For example, therapy clients often talk about the praise and comfort they received from a beloved teacher, mentor, or relative. When they feel alone or are struggling emotionally, the memory of the kind words spoken by this important person often help them to feel better.

Some of it depends on you. You teach yourself how to self-soothe through trial and error. For example, once on a particularly bad day, you may have pulled the covers over your head and stayed in bed. It seemed to help. More sleep calmed you down, and you woke up in a much better mood. So the next time you feel so stressed-out, you might try the same method. You also might have achieved some goals that help you to feel good about yourself, like running a marathon. When you're feeling down in the dumps, thinking about this accomplishment can help you to feel better about yourself.

If you don't have a strong set of skills already in place, this means it's important to work on developing them now. The good news, according to attachment theory, is that it is possible to strengthen these skills. This is one reason that people go into therapy, to learn (or relearn) the self-soothing skills needed to cope with stressful events. If your old ways are not adequate, you can learn new ways to comfort and soothe yourself.

the reasons why eating is soothing

In the absence of strong internal self-soothing skills, eating becomes a common substitute (Freeman and Gil 2004; Macht 2008; Spoor et al. 2007). There are a number of reasons why food takes on the role of comforter. We can't ignore the fact that people wouldn't use it if it didn't succeed at making them feel better. Here are some of the psychological and physiological reasons that explain why eating feels so good:

- **Biochemical changes in your body.** Some foods increase the amount of neurotransmitters in your brain or induce other biochemical changes that provide comfort. Often, this is why people are so drawn to chocolate. Chocolate raises the levels of serotonin and other chemicals that have mood-enhancing qualities (Parker, Parker, and Brotchie 2006). For example, you might feel more excited or alert because chocolate raises your blood sugar; it also has traces of caffeine. So eating can prompt physiological and biochemical reactions throughout your body that are psychologically pleasurable.

- **Conditioned emotions.** Certain foods are mentally linked with emotions. Think for a moment of the feelings that arise when you say the word "chocolate" to yourself. Anticipation? Joy? Bliss? Guilt? You may experience these emotions because that's what you think you're supposed to feel. That's because you've seen or heard the word paired with these emotional words in ads and in everyday conversations.

- **Celebration.** Eating is strongly intertwined with the notion of celebration and holidays. When we celebrate, we feel good.

- **Innate behavior.** We are not the only creatures who eat to find comfort. Some animals also turn to food to regulate their stress levels. For example, when rats are injected with stress hormones, they consume more sugar. One study suggests that like rats, we turn to comfort foods to help balance our stress hormones (Dallman et al. 2003).

- **Comfort foods.** Certain foods are more soothing than others, especially those high in fat and sugar (Wansink, Cheney, and Chan 2003). Comfort foods are edibles like mashed potatoes, macaroni and cheese, potato chips, and chicken casserole—anything that tastes good and is palatable to your senses. Often, comfort foods are strongly associated with childhood. They may remind you of your mom's cooking or food that was served at birthday parties when you were a kid. Frequently, comfort foods are carbohydrate rich, which is associated with sensations that make you feel full. And when you feel full, you feel comforted.

- **Diverting your attention from negative feelings.** Eating seems to take the edge off negative feelings because it distracts and diverts your attention away from whatever is bothering you (Heatherton and Baumeister 1991; Macht 2008). When you engage in another activity, such as eating, you aren't as aware of feeling bad. In addition, you might feel bad about your eating habits rather than allow yourself to feel bad about the issue that's really bothering you.

- **Interrupting boredom.** If you constantly need to be busy or you struggle with boredom, you may find eating an engaging task and therefore soothing. Finding food, thinking about what you want to eat, preparing it, and cleaning up take a lot of energy. These actions feel purposeful and seem to fill the time productively.

- **Conditioning.** Parents, often unintentionally, reinforce the connection between self-soothing and eating very early in a child's life. Using a bottle to pacify a crying baby is a prime example. Parents find it easier to use a bottle rather than rocking or singing to the infant because the bottle (or the breast) works so well. Fast-forward to this child as a toddler. Her mother gives the child a cookie to distract from the pain of a scraped knee. Again, food is associated with making the child feel better. If you treat yourself to a brownie to perk up your mood, it's likely that someone used food to console you in your past.

- **Dieting.** Dieters are particularly vulnerable to emotional eating (Polivy and Herman 2005). Emotional eating provides an immediately pleasurable reward rather than working toward the distant goal of becoming healthier and slimmer. It takes a lot of thought and energy to restrain one's eating. If you're stressed-out, it may be too demanding to find ways to reduce your food intake, which can lead to abandoning your diet plan.

- **Arousal.** Eating may feel good because it stimulates you. Low-arousal states, such as boredom, tend to increase food consumption. However, for some people, sadness and chronic stress are less likely to increase eating and may even lead to weight loss (Macht 2008; Polivy and Herman 2005).

- **Habit.** If you do anything repeatedly, it becomes a habit. Activities that feel familiar, even if they're unhealthy, can be soothing. For example, when you go on vacation and then return home, it's comforting to reenter your old routines, despite the fact that you would rather being sitting on the beach under a palm tree.

- **Modeling.** It's likely that you picked up your means of coping from your early caregivers or by observing the people around you. People tend to model the eating behaviors of their caregivers (Wardle et al. 2002). Maybe you watched your stressed-out mom dive into a bag of tortilla chips whenever she returned from visiting her supercritical aunt. Or perhaps a friend suggested going out for ice cream when you had the blues. You may have picked up the habit of eating to calm down by watching TV. Many TV commercials push the therapeutic value of food as a ploy to get you to buy their products.

So why is the soothing effect temporary and ultimately unsuccessful? It is difficult, even impossible sometimes, to eat just the right amount of food to feel truly comforted. Eating is pleasurable only up to a point. When you nibble past feeling full to feeling stuffed, comfort quickly turns to discomfort. Sometimes there is a time delay between the pleasure you feel while you are eating and the physiological reactions your body has after consuming and digesting the food, not to mention that the entertainment and pleasure value of eating wears off quickly. Snacking may distract you temporarily from your worries, but those underlying feelings come right back. For all of these reasons, the soothing qualities of food are often fleeting.

As you have seen, there are many reasons why eating feels soothing. Some of these reasons may seem familiar to you. If so, that's okay. While you read this book, keep in mind some of the specific reasons why you use food to comfort yourself.

when your self-soothing skills need a boost

Physical and emotional problems are likely to crop up in everyone's life, but if you know self-soothing skills, you are much better prepared to deal with them productively. Life is full of stress and responsibility. Most people need a way to calm down almost daily. That's why food is such an overly used self-soothing mechanism. You are seldom more than fifty feet away from some form of food at any moment, whether it's a vending machine or a fast-food restaurant. It is legal, cheap, and easy to get. The problems associated with using food to self-soothe range from merely annoying to life threatening.

- The guilt caused by overeating is both irritating and frustrating. My clients spend many sessions discussing the guilt and shame they feel due to repeating the same cycle over and over again. Regret, shame, and guilt can get in the way of being productive and enjoying life.

- Feeling too full from excess eating can make you feel sluggish, uncomfortable, or overweight.

- The temporary highs from eating followed by guilt or the original stress that caused you to overeat in the first place can be hard on your mood and damaging to your self-esteem.

- Overeating may lead to weight gain, which, in turn, can lead to many health complications and problems.

- When people have little or no ability to calm themselves down, in extreme cases they're in a constant state of disarray and internal chaos. Everything is a crisis. Friends and family members feel as though they are walking on eggshells around you, because your moods are intense and can be unpredictable. Unknowingly, you may become a threat to your most valued intimate relationships. You may take out your frustration on the person closest to you or place the burden of comforting you on his or her shoulders.

- Little or no ability to self-soothe in healthy ways is characteristic of a disorder called *borderline personality disorder*. People who have this disorder display a pattern of self-harm, such as chronic abuse of alcohol or hurting their bodies. Or they may damage their relationships because of their anger, or have inappropriate boundaries, which leads to them to push others away or to become too dependent on another person. Ironically, for some people, self-harm can actually be calming. It distracts from the original problem and places the pain directly under the person's control. It is that person's way of calming down, even it if it is potentially harmful.

- A number of clinical disorders are associated with problems of self-soothing. Addictive behaviors (drugs, alcohol, gambling), obsessive-compulsive disorder, obesity, anorexia, bulimia, and borderline personality disorder are but a few examples.

When your self-soothing skills are not well developed, this can be a major problem. Life is full of little hiccups and major hurdles. You have to find a healthy way to cope. If turning to food to alleviate stress sounds like you, don't worry. Practicing by using the tools provided in this book will help you begin to turn this around.

2 how to get started

The beginning is the most important part of the work.
—Plato

Okay, let's get ready. The urge to stress eat can hit at any time—today, tomorrow, next week. You have to get yourself prepared before it happens. Even when you know what to do when you're feeling blah, sometimes it's hard to get the ball rolling. Getting up off the couch or closing a box of cookies can be tough, even when you are fully aware that it will help. If this sounds like your current challenge, you can think about approaching this task in three different ways: you can mindfully change, take very small steps, or take a leap of faith. You can even combine these ways in a pattern that suits you.

mindfully change

You can observe a lot, just by watching.
—Yogi Berra

A mindful approach is a good way for most people to start a new behavior because it doesn't take a lot of effort. At first, you don't even have to change your behavior. Because of this, many people can easily commit to starting by using a mindful approach. Before you begin, remember that looking for nonfood alternatives to soothe yourself is an ongoing process. There is no pressure or hurry. Go at your own pace.

The first step is mindful observation. During this phase, don't try to avoid or cut down on your comfort eating. Your only task is to place all of your attention on your eating patterns and habits. For at least a week (or longer if you need extra time), just observe and keep track of what prompts you to seek food for comfort. Write down the signals that prompt you to eat. You can do this in a variety of ways, but the best way is to keep a journal while you're reading this book.

What circumstances make you the most vulnerable? Are there specific feelings? Do you do it at the same time each day? Simply watch yourself. Begin to understand your patterns. Think deeply about what you learn about yourself. You may be amazed that just by watching yourself closely, you can cut down on your emotional eating. This isn't really surprising. Think about how much harder you work when your boss is in the room with you. When no one is watching—even yourself—you may be less likely to utilize 100 percent of your efforts.

Once you have a better sense of why you seek food for comfort, it will be time to move on to the next phase: to live with more awareness. Pay close attention to your emotions and your body from moment to moment. As soon as you feel the urge to comfort yourself with food, gently acknowledge this feeling. Observe it without necessarily obeying it. Be sure to record the urge in your journal. Then read the mindfulness exercises in this book.

The mindful approach is helpful to many. Another way to get started is to ease into it with small steps.

take small steps

We cannot do everything at once, but we can do something at once. —Calvin Coolidge

Shaping is another way to approach behavior change. The method is to take baby steps toward the behavior you wish to adopt. For example, let's say that when you feel the need to emotionally eat, it would be helpful to pick up your journal and write about what's bothering you. You already know that using a healthy coping skill would be a better option than gobbling up snacks. But you just don't feel motivated to do it. You know what you want to do, but for some reason you can't seem to make it happen.

In such a situation, you may want to consider motivating yourself by shaping your behavior. *Shaping* is a behavior modification technique. It helps you adopt a new behavior by rewarding gradual steps that bring you closer to fully adopting the desired behavior. First, just focus on a behavior close to journaling. For example, pick up a scrap of paper. Jot down a few notes. You don't need full sentences. A few words or phrases will do. Any thoughts are a great start. You can always paste the scrap of paper into your journal later. You could even jot a few words down on your calendar.

After you do this small bit of writing, you may want to give yourself a small, nonfood reward. Rewarding yourself can be very reinforcing. *Reinforcement* is an effective way to increase a desired behavior. You don't always need a tangible reward, such as a new lipstick, a magazine, or a cup of coffee. For instance, you can give yourself permission to sleep in ten more minutes in the morning or to relax in a bubble bath. Sometimes effective reinforcement comes from feeling good about just starting to work on a goal.

Right now, the important point to understand is that you don't have to do any of the self-soothing methods perfectly. Just do something close to the behavior you want to acquire to get the ball rolling. If taking baby steps is too slow for you, try the approach described next, taking a leap of faith.

a leap of faith

Stop talking. Start walking. —L. M. Heroux

A leap of faith is the jump-right-in approach; it means to fully engage in the desired behavior right off the bat. You don't do it gradually. You do it all at once. The idea is that the more you expose yourself to the new skill you want to acquire, the more you become habituated to it; that is, the more you get used to it. It becomes less foreign, more comfortable, and easier to do when you need to practice it.

In the case of self-soothing, jumping headfirst into a new soothing behavior may be the best option for many people. We often wait too long for something to feel right, when actually it will feel comfortable only after we've done it for a while. So at first it may feel unnatural or uncomfortable using the new ways to soothe yourself described in this book. In fact, it may feel just plain weird.

Let's return to the journaling example mentioned above. But in this case, instead of slowly easing yourself into writing, you get out your journal immediately. Then you commit to writing for ten minutes—even if you don't feel like it. Most of the time, after you get started, you're glad you did. Exercising is often described this way. Many people say that they never feel like going to the gym. Nevertheless, after an hour of working out, they feel great and are happy they went. With time, using your new ways of soothing yourself will become a routine habit, like exercising.

When you pass up the opportunity to soothe yourself with food, give yourself as much praise as possible. You may even want to tell a friend, a family member, or anyone who will ooh and aah over your newfound skills. You might consider rewarding yourself for doing the right thing. Remember, you are working on diminishing the emotionally rewarding aspect of eating.

To help turn the techniques into habits, make a chart with a list of the self-soothing tips you would like to try. Keep track of your successes. Write down praise for your efforts. If you are someone who needs something more tangible than words, paste a little sticker next to your new behavior each time you engage in it.

Jumping right in will help you to see that new ways of comforting yourself are not as bad as you might have thought they would be. And your list will aid you in turning them into new habits. Trying to think in these ways can help you to stop avoiding.

getting organized

Which approach will work best for you? That depends. To answer that question, you must know yourself well. If you aren't sure, this section will help you figure it out. And even if you do know what will work for you, it's important to get organized, just as if you were packing for a trip. Investing a small amount of time in preparing to use the self-soothing techniques in this book will help the process go smoothly. There are two important steps:

1. **Check in with yourself.** If you are currently struggling with emotional eating, every morning when you get up, take a minute to check in with yourself and do a self-soothing forecast for the day. This is a bit like getting the weather report and using it to choose your clothing for the day. If it's cold, you'll bring a sweater. If it's likely to be a stormy day, you need to bring the right rain gear to deal with the difficulties you will meet. If the forecast for self-

soothing looks rough, toss your journal into your bag. Bring along the phone number of someone you may want to call later. Take this book to read as a quick pick-me-up or to strengthen your motivation.

2. **Take an inventory.** Before you get started, take an inventory of your current self-soothing skills. It's likely that you've developed some methods naturally that succeed in calming you down. For example, instead of eating, you might take a nap or spend some time alone doing a self-soothing activity.

Take a moment now to list your strengths and most successful soothing activities. Sometimes we get too focused on the skills that we lack and forget about those we have. If you aren't sure of what your self-soothing skills are, remember the last time you had a bad day. What did you do to make yourself feel better? Write down all the non-food-related ways you use to cope with a bad mood. As you read this book, keep in mind how you can capitalize on or enhance your natural skills. Perhaps you will weave the new skills you'll learn in this book into some of the techniques you're already using.

is it emotional or physical hunger?
How to Tell the Difference

If you aren't sure whether you want to eat because you're truly hungry or because your emotions need calming and soothing, do a quick self-check before starting to eat. Ask yourself if any of the following statements describe your hunger. Then add up how many times you agree with these statements. Observe whether you agree with more statements under emotional hunger or belly hunger.

Emotional Hunger

Emotional hunger is characterized by some or all of the following behaviors:

- Your desire to eat comes on quickly and intensely like an on/off switch. Your degree of hunger can go from zero to ten in a matter of moments.

- You are very open to suggestion (for example, a coworker says she's going out for a donut, and suddenly a donut sounds very good to you).

- Your hunger increases with certain feelings, particularly stress.

- You can't think through your options. Your feeling of hunger is so intense that you don't care what your options are—until after you have eaten something.

- Your hunger is such that it urges you to engage in mindless eating—that is, not really tasting your food or eating it in an automatic, mechanical way (for example, mindlessly popping a packet of M&M's into your mouth one by one).

- You crave a particular kind of food, like chocolate or fast-food; something that would be merely filling just won't do.

- A sense of satisfaction is hard to reach, and it seems unrelated to how full or how empty your stomach is.

- You often have the fleeting thought before you begin eating that you may feel guilty after you've eaten. Also, you often experience guilt after you finish eating.

Belly Hunger

True physical hunger is related to blood sugar levels. Therefore, your physical need for food is based on what and when you ate last.

- You notice that your need for food grows gradually in accordance with the time and the number of meals you ate. For example, between breakfast and lunch your hunger increases at a slowly rising rate.

- You are looking for something filling, and you're open to many different options to fill that hunger, rather than craving a specific taste.

- You experience distinct physiological hunger cues, like a rumbling stomach. In the extreme, you may feel grouchy or even get a headache.

- You tend to quit eating when you are full.

- Your awareness of your body's changing sensations as you move from hunger to satiety while you are eating, creates a sense of satisfaction.

- You know that feeding your physical hunger is essential as the fuel that nourishes you and keeps you going.

- You can wait a while to eat, instead of needing to eat compulsively at the very moment you feel the urge or desire to eat.

- Your hunger is not in any way associated with guilt. You know that you need to eat and you feel okay about eating.

If you agreed with more statements under emotional hunger than under belly hunger, then you would benefit more from a self-soothing technique than from reaching for a snack.

3 mindful meditation techniques

Mindful meditation techniques are great for helping you get through strong urges to emotionally eat. Note that these skills don't completely erase the craving or emotional discomfort. Unfortunately, such erasure is impossible. If you were able to banish all food cravings from your life, you would have already done so. However, mindfulness skills can help you ride the urge out until the desire to emotionally eat fades or goes away.

As discussed in the introduction, *being mindful* is a way of thinking. Basically, it is being very aware of the present moment in an open and nonjudgmental way. Many people are drawn to food for unconscious reasons. When they slow down and really pay attention to whatever triggers their craving for food, especially when they aren't hungry, they get a better handle on how to deal with their cravings.

Your task in this chapter is to use the power of your mind to become very aware of your urges to eat—in new ways. Stop mentally pushing your cravings away and beating yourself up for using food as a tranquilizer. Instead, embrace your yearning for food. Get to know it. Investigate it in a curious but uncritical way. This may sound counterintuitive. But when you do this, you will understand why you need comfort. Only then can you choose the precisely right calming activity that will soothe you just as well, if not better, than food.

1. creating mindful moments

Sometimes I am so busy rushing from one thing to another that I am not even aware of what I am doing or feeling. I unconsciously pop chocolate kisses or M&M's into my mouth. Later, after it's too late, I realize I was nibbling on food because I was worried and upset. When I'm mindful, I enjoy life more because I am really present as things are happening, not just analyzing things later. Being more aware has also taught me how to recognize when I am mindlessly eating simply to comfort myself. —Kelly

Kelly mindlessly munches on a bowl of potato chips. It's her Sunday night ritual. Thinking about Monday morning and the rest of her upcoming week leads to half an hour of stress eating. Time flies by as she nibbles and slips into a trancelike state. Suddenly she jolts out of it and realizes that she has polished off the entire bowl. But she didn't really taste one bite. Eating automatically in a robotic way is a familiar act for her and it creates a familiar feeling. Sometimes Kelly gets so caught up worrying while she's driving that she heads to work instead of to the grocery store as she had intended. The same kind of zoning out happens when she thinks about her kids while she reads a novel. She can't remember anything she just read.

For emotional eaters like Kelly, routine activities, such as eating, provide a prime opportunity to slip into a different state of consciousness. Focusing only on your thoughts and tuning out other sensations happening in your body can make you very vulnerable to stress eating. You are likely to lose track of why you are eating or how much you plan to eat. Emotional eating may have become such a habit in your daily life that you might find yourself slipping into it without even realizing that you are doing it.

The antidote to doing things on autopilot whether it is reading, driving, or stress eating is to do all of your activities with full awareness. Be mindful of your body and its sensations at all times, instead of allowing your mind take over. If you are driving, notice how the steering wheel feels in your hands. If you are reading, listen to the sound of the page as it turns. To avoid stress eating, be in the moment. If you feel at risk of engaging in stress eating, play close attention to what your body is doing. For example, direct your attention to the placement of your hands. How do they feel? Are they cold? Where are they resting? Noticing your sensations you will help you to stay engaged with what your body is feeling and doing rather than allowing your hand to grab food automatically for comfort.

Practice bringing mindfulness to the routine activities you do every day, such as brushing your teeth, washing the dishes, or riding a bike. It's likely you do these things so often that they are done automatically. Instead of doing these activities in an automatic way, bring your full awareness to them. Notice the bubbles and scent of the soap as you wash dishes. Focus on your hands' circular motions. Be mentally present and focused on every action and sensation.

How can you step away from thoughts that keep urging you to eat? The mindful answer is to direct your focus away from your thoughts and onto your body. Place your attention on whatever your body is doing and feeling—like walking or stretching, or how the warm dishwater feels on your hands. The following exercise will tell you more specifically how to do this.

~self-soothing technique~
Stop and Mindfully Smell the Roses

It's likely that an ordinary walk would be a helpful activity to substitute for stress eating. But you might want to try taking a mindful walk. Not only will this get your mind on something other than food, it will also help you to calm down and center yourself.

How does a mindful walk differ from an ordinary walk? Well, as you stroll, notice the scenery. Look around. Don't power walk. Bring your attention to the feeling of your feet hitting the ground. Close your eyes for a moment. Turn your attention to what you hear. Then open your eyes and look closely at everything around you. Use all of your senses. Observe what you see as if you were describing the scene to someone who was blindfolded. Tune in to your body and what it does during this walk. Can you feel your heartbeat? How is your breathing? When you quiet the chatter of your mind and focus on your sensations, you will become a little calmer. The next time you have the urge to emotionally eat, don't just go for a stroll—go for a mindful walk.

~self-soothing technique~
Count on Your Senses 5-4-3-2-1

When you have trouble clearing your mind of thoughts of food, try focusing on your senses.

1. State one scent you can smell.

2. Name two sounds you can hear.

3. Describe three sensations your body is feeling, such as temperature, the texture of your sweater, your feet against the ground.

4. Identify four colors that you see.

5. To yourself, begin by naming five things you see in front of you.

When you finish doing this, it's likely that you will be thinking about nothing, not even food—unless there's food directly in front of you. If you are still thinking about food, repeat each step until you notice that your thoughts are less clouded by food cravings.

2. the practice of meditating

Food. Food. Food. I think about food a lot. When I start
thinking about all of the desserts that sound good to eat, suddenly
I can't get sweets and chocolate off my mind. Thoughts like
these keep going around in my brain like a merry-go-round.
Meditation is the only thing that helps me make mental peace
with food. —John

You've probably tried several tricks to get the cheesecake in the
back of the refrigerator out of your mind: ignored it, tried to
pretend it wasn't there, pleaded with yourself, or tried to talk
yourself out of wanting it. But emptying your mind of thoughts
filled with food is no easy task.

The good news is that meditation is a helpful technique for
clearing your mind, even when it is stuck on food. Meditating
helps you look deeply into the origin of your food cravings. It
makes your mind seem like a still lake. When your mind is placid
and serene, you can see to the bottom. When it is active with
painful and turbulent emotions, it's hard to see what's below the
surface or what might be causing the turbulence.

Meditation may seem hokey or just the latest, trendy new age
fad. But it isn't. It is thousands of years old, and is simply a way
to calm yourself down by helping you to regulate your body's
natural *fight-or-flight response*. This physiological response occurs
when you are stressed. Your body gets ready to fight or flee,
which increases your heart rate and adrenaline flow, slows your
digestive processes, constricts your blood vessels, and quickens
your breathing. Meditation tones down this response by induc-

ing its opposite: the relaxation response. The *relaxation response* reverses the fight-or-flight response by slowing down your heart rate and breathing, lowering your blood pressure, and relaxing your muscles.

One of the nicest things about meditation is that it's free and easy to do, and you can do it anywhere. Meditation provides many psychological and physical benefits (Baer 2003; Brown, Ryan, and Creswell 2007; Davidson et al. 2003; Shapiro et al. 2008).

Psychological Benefits of Meditation

- Reduces stress and anxiety

- Increases self-esteem

- Decreases irritability and moodiness

- Increases calmness

- Increases ability to concentrate and focus

Physical Benefits of Meditation

- Creates a relaxation response in the body, slowing the heart and respiratory rates

- Increases serotonin levels, which is helpful because low levels of serotonin are linked with depression, anxiety, obesity and headaches

- Decreases production of stress hormones

- Improves sleep

- Increases energy levels

- Increases immunity to illness

As you can see, these psychological and physical benefits are the perfect medicine for the emotional eater.

~self-soothing technique~
Meditation Styles

There are many different meditation styles (or techniques). When you can't stop obsessing about food or need relief, try one of the following techniques. See which one fits your personality and is the most helpful for you.

Concentration Meditation

One way to meditate is to concentrate all of your attention on a single point. This point can be an image or an object. Begin by sitting quietly and focusing all of your attention on this object. Really look at it. Describe it to yourself. It is often helpful to focus on a detail, such as part of an image or the tip of a candle flame. The closer you look at it, the more likely it is that you will see something you didn't notice at first.

Brooke, for example, is a frequent emotional eater. She counters her emotional eating by focusing on a photograph of Paris in her living room, rather than staying in the kitchen. When she starts to feel the need to stress eat, she firmly plants herself within inches of this picture and focuses all of her attention on the top point of the Eiffel Tower. This is a little like zooming in with a camera. She narrows her consciousness to include only this image rather than the images of food that had been swirling around in her mind. If thoughts of food are generated, she gently acknowledges the thought to herself, and then says good-bye to it. Then she redirects her focus to the meditation point. She continues doing this for however long it takes to calm herself.

Mantra Meditation

In mantra meditation, you focus on a sound or sounds. *Mantras* are intended to channel your thoughts away from any negative self-talk going on in your mind. The statements that keep you stuck, such as "I can't stand feeling this way!" are *negative self-talk*. A mantra can be a sound, a word, a phrase, or even a sentence. But how does focusing on a mantra help the emotional eater?

It helps by actively controlling the focus of your attention to be on calming words. This focus is a complete contrast to following the random thoughts that pop into your head, which often encourage you to eat; thoughts like "I must have a candy bar right now!"

To begin, close your eyes and repeat a sound or phrase. Say it out loud. In the Hindi language, "om" is described as the vibration of all living things. Notice how it feels to shape your lips as you push out the sound. Notice how your body and lips vibrate as you make the sound. If you don't like this or it doesn't work for you, try more familiar sounds or words. You can use words or phrases like "peace," "I'm okay," "Allow it to be," "love," and "I'm open to what is."

When you repeat the mantra several times in a row, you will find that your mind focuses and you can concentrate on creating the sound. If you are thinking about your bank balance or any other worries, it is hard to continue repeating or chanting the mantra. But it is worth the effort. Essentially, mantras help to quiet the inner dialogue that is likely adding to your stress. When the dialogue has been quieted, you can think more rationally about food, and then explore the best way to comfort and soothe yourself.

Mindfulness Meditation

This type of meditation involves observing and paying attention to your thoughts and emotions. You turn your attention toward, not away from, your thoughts, as you do with concentration meditation. From closely examining how you think and why you're thinking about food, you get a better understanding of the emotions you're trying to soothe. If you discover what's really bothering you, you can determine a more effective way to calm yourself.

Give yourself one minute to do this exercise. If you need more, that's okay. But begin by committing to just one minute. Stop what you are doing. Sit quietly. Direct all of your attention to your thoughts. Then just observe your thoughts swimming around in your mind. Breathe deeply. Close your eyes if it helps you to focus.

Now think of a time when you recently overate. Or you can try this when you are experiencing an emotional food craving. You will be just observing, in a nonjudgmental way, the thoughts and feelings you have about this desire.

To help with this meditation, you can imagine that you are a bystander at a parade watching from a distance. Each thought you have is on its own parade float. Perhaps you have thoughts like "I need chocolate! Why shouldn't I eat it? I'm such a failure at eating healthy anyway." Imagine that these thoughts are written on one float. Watch the float as it approaches you, passes by, and disappears in the distance. Allow your thoughts and feelings be whatever they are. Too often, we try to stop or change our thoughts by telling ourselves, "Stop thinking that!"

Instead, ask yourself with a gentle and open curiosity, "I'm wondering why I think I need chocolate to feel better? What happened today that would make that thought enter my mind?" Now imagine placing the next thought that follows that one onto the next float. Observe what kind of thoughts continue to parade through your mind. Are they guilty? Irrational? Angry? Observing individual thoughts slows down your automatic thought processes. It also helps you to observe yourself from a distance so that you get less caught up in the content of your thoughts.

3. breathe your way to inner calm

When I realize that I'm stress eating and I just can't calm down, I take a few deep breaths. It seems to clean out all the negative feelings and stops me from scarfing down another bowl of ice cream. —Michele

Michele lay awake most nights worrying about everything she could possibly think of: from the trivial, like wondering if she'd turned off the light in the kitchen, to larger worries, like the possibility that her mother's health was declining. Late-night munching seemed to help her relax and let go of her anxieties. Unfortunately, after a few minutes of distracting herself with cookies and milk, the same old worries came roaring back, topped with guilt feelings and a stomach that felt uncomfortably full. However, Michele discovered that mindful breathing exercises were the perfect antidote to stress eating for her.

Mindful breathing may be a helpful skill for you to learn too. Does it seem odd that something you do every single minute of your life can also be healing and therapeutic? Mindful breathing draws your attention away from troubling thoughts and stressful feelings. Instead of focusing on the content of the words in your mind instructing you to get food *now*, you direct your attention to a very different monologue. You talk to yourself about how to breathe well.

Try this for a moment. After you read these instructions, put down the book. Turn your attention to your breathing. Describe to yourself how you are taking in air—fast, slow, shallow, or holding your breath. Pay attention to how your breathing changes when you are actively thinking about this automatic behavior. Once you have done this, note how your attention shifts to your body. Your mind momentarily moves away from whatever you were thinking about to notice what is going on in your body. Simply practicing these instructions disengages your mind from thinking about food, even if it is only for a few moments.

Thankfully, you don't have to think about taking each breath. Breathing is a bodily function that happens automatically. Your body is programmed to make it happen all on its own. The interesting aspect about breathing is that you can override the automatic system. You can make your breathing go faster, or you can slow it down. You can take over the driver's seat.

Being able to control your breathing can be used to your advantage. You can trick your body into believing that you are resting or going to sleep. This will prepare your body to relax rather than eat. If your body thinks it's going to be fed, it will start producing saliva so that you can chew food. This physiological response moves you one step closer to eating. On the other hand, if your body thinks you are about to relax or go to sleep, it sends the appropriate signals to slow down throughout your body.

Mindful breathing also can increase the oxygen flow in your body, which helps you to think more clearly. Rational thinking helps you come up with good alternatives to soothing yourself with cupcakes and leftover macaroni and cheese.

If you aren't convinced yet that breathing exercises have healing powers, consider the Lamaze breathing exercises used for coping with the pain of natural childbirth. If breathing exercises can help women cope with the level of pain that comes with birthing a child, they can surely help you with whatever emotional turmoil you're experiencing.

~self-soothing technique~
Breathing Exercises

Sometimes people are afraid of breathing exercises because they fear that doing them takes a long time. They don't need to be long. They can be as long or as short as you would like them to be. As an added bonus, you can do them anywhere, anytime; for example, while you are driving, waiting for your order at a restaurant, or sitting in your own living room. Choose an exercise to match your mood from those listed below.

Here are some tips: Try doing these breathing exercises when you aren't feeling stressed or aren't smack dab in the middle of emotional eating. Note that it takes a lot of practice to get their full benefits. Don't give up. Also, expect your mind to wander away and become distracted during these exercises. That's inevitable. When this happens, just keep bringing your mind back to the task at hand.

Calming breath. This is good for emotional eaters who turn to food to pacify strong feelings. Use this technique when you feel short of breath, anxious, or out of control:

1. Start with relaxing your neck and shoulder muscles.

2. Breathe in slowly through your nose, and as you inhale count to three.

3. Pretend that you're going whistle.

4. Breathe out through pursed lips, letting the air out naturally. You don't have to change your breathing or force the air out of your lungs.

5. Bring to mind the image of blowing bubbles.

6. Repeat. Keep doing pursed-lip breathing until you feel calmer.

Relaxing breath. This is good for those emotional eaters who seek food when they are trying to relax and unwind:

1. Sit or stand, whichever is more comfortable for you.

2. Close your eyes if you want to.

3. Bend your arms at the elbows. Pull your elbows toward each other behind your back. Stretch your elbows back behind you as far as they will go.

4. Hold for a moment, then let your arms drop by your sides.

5. Inhale deeply.

6. Hold your breath as you count to three.

7. Exhale slowly.

8. Let all the air out.

9. Repeat steps 3 through 6 as many times as it takes to feel more relaxed.

Cleansing breath. This works well for overeaters who need to clear out negative thoughts or worries:

1. Sit or stand comfortably.

2. Inhale slowly and deeply through your nose.

3. Hold that breath for a few seconds.

4. Pretend that you have a straw in your mouth and exhale a short burst of air forcefully through the small opening. Blow the entire breath out in little spurts of air. With each puff out, visualize blowing away any pollutants, toxic thoughts, or worries, continuing until you've emptied your lungs via these short, strong puffs. Imagine all of your toxic thoughts and worries falling into a puddle on the floor.

5. Repeat steps 2 through 4 six to ten times.

Energizing breath. This works well for overeaters who turn to food for quick energy, to procrastinate, or when they're bored:

1. Stand comfortably.

2. Raise and extend your arms straight up into the air three times. Then lower them.

3. Each time you do this, extend your arms a little further into the air.

4. Turn your attention to your breathing.

5. Breathe deeply. Your breathing can be natural. It doesn't have to be altered.

6. Extend your arms out to your sides at shoulder height, then rotate them in the air ten times, circling up and then back.

7. Reverse directions, circling your arms down and then back ten times.

8. If you need an image to focus on, imagine your arms as a windmill.

One-minute mindful breathing. Remind yourself to breathe deeply often. Write "breathe deeply" on a Post-it note and paste it on your bathroom mirror. Put another note on your computer monitor and put some more notes in other places where you will see them often. Send yourself an e-mail or text message to breathe deeply. Do whatever you have to do to remember to practice this energizing breath.

4. strengthen your endurance to counter stress eating

I love blueberry cake donuts. I even dream about them in my sleep. Today, I was totally stressed-out. I thought I would treat myself to one. Maybe I'd feel a little bit better. I ate one. Nothing. I ate another. Nothing. Five donuts later, I felt terrible. Why didn't I stop after the first donut? Why didn't just one make me feel better if that's what they really do? —Sarah

The skill of mindful observation can be very helpful for dealing with what some of my clients call the "emotional food scavenger" within them. Emotional food scavengers search for a good thing to eat until something is found that will hit the spot. They hope that if they find the right or perfect food, they'll feel satisfied or better. The scavenger's intent is to feel soothed and calmed rather than quieting a hungry belly. The emotional food scavenger is hungry, but not for food.

The real question is, what is the emotional hunger for? Are you lonely? Stressed? Nervous? What is eating covering up or numbing out for you? If you knew the answer, you could discover what would really make you feel better. A donut can't even begin to fill your need for connection. Calling a friend can be the best antidote to loneliness. That's why it's essential to be more mindful of what your urge to eat is trying to tell you.

To answer the question of what you really need, try slowing down and responding to this urge to eat instead of merely reacting to it. At this point in your life, eating to soothe yourself has become like a knee-jerk reaction. You feel the urge to emotionally eat, and then you obey this internal desire quickly and automatically. So, how can you slow yourself down to get to the heart of your need for comfort?

~self-soothing technique~
Minding the Emotional Gap

Respond mindfully to your hunger. Work on consciously choosing how you will calm yourself rather than following automatic and habitual patterns. To do this, it is often helpful to create a gap between feeling hunger and responding to it. Your task in this exercise is to lengthen the time interval, the gap, between noticing your hunger and responding to it. It is likely to be between five and ten minutes. Such an interval gives you time to explore your options and consciously decide what you want to do: act on the urge to stress eat, or do something other than eat.

If your urge to eat is really emotional rather than physical, your desire to eat will fade when you find something to do that will distract you from food. When your mind is fully focused on something else, time flies by unnoticed. You've probably also noticed how your emotions change dramatically over time. Observe how your urge to eat will lose its intensity with the passage of time if it isn't based on real hunger.

Aim to lengthen the time gap between noticing your hunger and responding to it. Begin by checking in with your body. Label the level of your emotional hunger from 1 to 10, with 10 meaning the strongest urge to eat. Your task in this exercise is to lengthen the time interval, the gap, between noticing your hunger and responding to it. If you can extend it to five to ten minutes, this will give you time to explore your options.

~self-soothing technique~
Try a Quick Breathing Exercise

In this technique, you work on coping with the urge to emotionally eat one moment at a time. The urge can become overwhelming if you think that you'll have to endure your strong desire without responding to it for a longer period of time, such as an hour or two. It feels much more manageable when you focus on coping only one moment at a time. You can do one minute of anything.

- Redirect the content of your thoughts from "Must eat now" to more positive, affirming thoughts that encourage you to allow the urge to come and go. Focus on coping one moment at a time. You may find your mind fights this process by saying, "Oh, that won't work." Such thoughts will keep you stuck. Instead, say to yourself, "I will try."

- On your in-breath, inhale slowly and say a phrase that reflects your strength and fortitude. Say one of these phrases to yourself: "I'm resilient," "I can do this," "I'm okay without food," or "I will survive."

- On your out-breath, exhale slowly and say a sentence indicating that this feeling will change. Use sentences like "I'm waiting patiently for it to end," "I can hang in here," "This isn't forever," or "I can take it one moment at a time."

- Commit to doing this for one minute. At the end of that one minute, check in with your body. Where is your level of emotional hunger on a scale of 1 to 10 now?

- Ask yourself if you can commit to one more minute of doing this exercise.

- The strength of your urge to eat will either fall or be lessened a little, even if only a tiny amount. You will build your confidence that you will be okay if you don't obey the urge to numb out or obtain pleasure from food.

If you have trouble focusing on your breathing, fill the gap between noticing your hunger and responding to it with mindful observations. Count the number of tiles on the floor or the ceiling. Or find and name everything in the room that is blue. You can also try some of your own ideas about ways to fill the gap. Then reassess the level of your emotional hunger from 1 to 10.

5. letting go

I yelled at myself for ordering a greasy appetizer at dinner. I didn't need it and I just blew my diet. I told myself for the hundredth time, "Just let it go!" The rational side of my brain knew this was the best plan. But there is nothing I can do about that now. When I get something in my head, I can't seem to let go of it. —Samantha

Letting go is an act in which you release your need to control the situation. You stop telling yourself how it should be and begin focusing on dealing with how things really are right now. This attitude allows you to open up to new insights. When you see issues as they really are, you can start finding new ways to address them.

Letting go of, or not responding to, an urge to emotionally eat can take some practice. Samantha, a thirty-one-year-old high school teacher, felt strongly compelled to act on her every craving. She couldn't allow thoughts of food to exit from her mind. Sometimes she literally found herself unable to put down her bowl of breakfast cereal until she either felt better emotionally or the contents of the entire cereal box were completely gone. When this happened, she felt overstuffed and very uncomfortable. Then she became angry at herself and found other ways to beat herself up emotionally.

Emotional eaters may discover that they have trouble letting go of many things, not just their guilt over their mindless eating episodes. Holding on to something that upsets or angers you is often more harmful to you than the event that triggered your anger in the first place. Also, stewing about things you just can't change can be a powerful trigger for emotional eating.

~self-soothing technique~
The Catch and Release Method

Letting go of stressful thoughts and food cravings is a little like catch and release fishing. Unlike traditional fishing, in which the fish is caught and kept, the catch and release method has you carefully unhook the fish and immediately throw it right back into the water. The trick is to do it quickly, without harming the fish. This is a good analogy for catching and releasing your thoughts. If a distressing thought is bothering you or your mind is stuck on wanting to eat, imagine yourself casting out a fishing line, catching that thought, reeling it in, and then releasing it right away.

This method is more soothing than trying to just ignore your hunger. When you try to push away your thoughts about specific foods or your desire to stress eat, a mental power struggle occurs. Take out the power struggle by gently recognizing that, yes, your urge to emotionally eat has been activated. Then deal with that by using the following dialogue as a model for your own internal dialogue.

Practice Dialogue

Catch: I need to find something to eat.

Release: Oh, there goes a thought about food.

Catch: Mmmm. I wonder what kind of leftovers I could heat up.

Release: Just because I'm thinking I need food doesn't mean that I have to eat.

Catch: You don't need it! You shouldn't be snacking, you pig!

Release: That was a judgmental thought.

Catch: Why am I so hard on myself?

Release: A thought is just a thought, I don't have to buy it.

~self-soothing technique~
Squeeze Bubble Wrap

If you find yourself eating because you are angry or you need to let go of or release a strong emotion, popping bubble wrap can be very therapeutic. The pressure needed to squeeze the plastic and the noise the squeezed plastic makes can be cathartic.

~self-soothing technique~
Skipping Emotional Stones

You can do this exercise beside the shore of a body of water such as an ocean, lake, river, or stream. (If you don't have a lake or stream nearby, use your imagination.) Gather a pile of small, relatively flat rocks that fit comfortably in your palm. Then skip each rock across the surface of the water. To do this, you throw the rock as if it were a Frisbee, but you throw it parallel to the water so that it skims the surface. If done correctly, you will see it bounce across the water. Each rock can represent a feeling. Imagine casting away the feeling that's disturbing you.

~self-soothing technique~
Letting-Go Breath

When you have trouble letting go of your desire to eat or you are flooded with negative thoughts or feelings that haunt you, try this next exercise:

1. Take three deep, slow breaths.

2. Reposition your body. It's very likely that your body has unconsciously taken a position that reflects what you are currently feeling. For example, if you are depressed, you might be hunched over. It's important to change your body position to help you let go of that feeling. If you were sitting, stand up.

3. Shake your entire body. Shake your hands, shoulders, arms, hips, buttocks, and thighs.

4. As you move, say to yourself, "I am letting go of whatever is happening."

5. Imagine thoughts falling away from you while you are shaking your entire body.

6. Take three more deep, slow breaths.

7. Repeat three more times.

6. setting the inner critic straight

"You are such an idiot! You are so fat! How could you eat that?" Unfortunately, these are some of the tamer thoughts I have. If I really told people the names I call myself when I overeat or give in to a craving, you'd be shocked. I'd never call my worst enemy some of these names. —Michele

Nothing sparks stress eating more than your own negative self-judgments. Sometimes it isn't your spouse or even your boss who makes you furious. It's your very own inner critic that has you all snarling and snapping. Soothing with food seems like your only lifeline. Ice cream and chocolate cake don't judge you, you do.

This inner critic can kick off a vicious cycle. Your self-criticism leads to shame and guilt, so you turn to food to pacify your critical feelings. But then you judge yourself again for wanting food, and the cycle begins again. Note that it's self-criticism of your own behavior that sometimes keeps the cycle going. The trick is to notice but not listen to your inner critic. Give yourself a gentle little nudge each time you become aware that your inner critic is speaking up.

If you use food to drown out the harsh judgments of your inner critic, it's helpful to have compassion. To have compassion for yourself means to be kind, nonjudgmental, and empathetic toward yourself. This mind-set allows you to be honest with yourself. When you hold back your judgments, you're more open to understanding why you feel the way you do. On the other hand, self-criticism causes you to avoid or shut down your thoughts. Compassion for yourself helps you understand the soothing that emotional eating gives you.

~self-soothing technique~
Compassion Meditation

Start practicing being compassionate by using the ancient technique of loving-kindness meditation. This is a well-known form of meditation that dates back thousands of years. Doing even a few minutes of this meditation has been shown to strengthen your sense of connection with others and increase positive feelings (Hutcherson, Seppala, and Gross 2008).

You start by directing kind words and thoughts toward yourself. While you say these words, remember that you deserve this kind of care. Then direct your compassion toward others. This includes all those whom you are close to. Then direct your compassion to the whole world. Initially, this may feel artificial or uncomfortable. You may not be accustomed to thinking about people you don't know. You may not know how to talk to yourself without criticizing. It will get easier with repetition. Here is the basic technique for sending loving-kindness to yourself:

1. Begin by sitting comfortably. Choose a quiet place away from the kitchen and other distractions. Relax. Allow your mind to settle and quiet down. Repeat the following statements silently in your mind or say them aloud if that helps.

May I be at peace with myself.

May I know joy with myself and eating.

May I be relaxed and well.

May I feel love for myself and my body.

May I find peace and calmness within myself, instead of seeking it in food.

(You may add any other phrase that feels important to you.)

2. First direct the statements toward yourself.

3. The next time you say them, direct your statements to a good friend. For example: May my friend Jessica be at peace with herself.

4. Then direct them to a neutral person (like an acquaintance).

5. Then send them to a difficult person.

6. Finally, send your phrases to the entire universe.

7. calmness, be right here, right now

I'm driving in my car. It's a gorgeous day and I'm as happy as can be. A song comes on the radio that reminds me of my ex-husband. It's the song we danced to at our wedding. I start to reminisce about my wedding day, and I think about my best friend, who was my maid of honor. She is now married to my ex-husband. In an instant, I'm seething mad. My knuckles whiten as I grip the steering wheel. It doesn't matter that this happened ten years ago or that I am happily remarried now. What's crazy is that nothing changed from five minutes ago except my thoughts. Mentally, I rehash all the events that led to the divorce. When I get home, I haven't calmed down and I pace around. I open the pantry door even though I'm not really hungry. I need to chew on something—anything—to stop thinking about my ex-husband and my ex-best friend! —Jane

Jane's process demonstrates the complex relationship between thoughts and emotional eating. Dwelling on past mistakes and regrets or trying to mentally rework them can send you straight into an emotional feeding frenzy. This is exactly what happened to Jane. Her mind traveled away from the present moment to dwell on past events she couldn't change. Just stewing over her past caused her enough distress to trigger emotional eating.

Focusing on the present—her happy remarriage and how she felt in the moment—would have helped Jane take charge of her emotional eating. Her first marriage might be over, but her emotional eating was happening right now. The only thing that she does have command over is her ability to change that very moment.

You can drive yourself crazy obsessing about unchangeable aspects of the past or worrying about a future you cannot control. In addition, when your mind drifts into long-ago moments, it's easy to zone out and mindlessly munch away. Keeping your mind anchored in the present, what is happening in the here and now can help you to remain calm.

~self-soothing technique~
Staying in the Present Moment

If you obsess on the past or worry about the future, try bringing your thoughts back to this very moment. Here are some ideas about how to do this:

- Anchor your mind to the room. If you need a visual image, imagine dropping a heavy anchor on the floor. Visualize the anchor at your feet. Don't allow your mind to drift with away from the room in which you are doing this.

- Did you every play the game I Spy when you were a child? It's a simple game. You say, "I spy something blue." Then your partner looks around trying to spot the blue object. To keep your mind from traveling into the past or future or to a painful place, try to stay in the room emotionally. You can do this just by being aware of what's happening in the room at this very moment. Play I Spy with all of your senses. Notice what you see, hear, and smell in the room. Notice the temperature in the room, the texture of the carpet, and the color of the wall. Focus only on what is happening within the four walls of the room.

- Try closing your eyes and repeating the words "here" and "now." Repeat these words several times.

8. mindful spiritual moments

Prayer is my main form of meditation. If I can't stop stress eating, I say a quick prayer asking for the strength to get through it without completely sabotaging myself. It helps me feel less alone and calms me down. It comforts me to know there is another power, stronger than I am, helping me get through this. I can't do it alone. —Mary

Mary went to France for six months on a study-abroad program. She loved her classes, but after three months she began struggling with homesickness. France was an easy place to get sucked in to emotional eating. On every corner, there was a crepe stand or a charcouterie bursting with fresh baguettes and rich cheeses for sale. If she kept on eating at this rate, she'd never fit into her travel clothing when she was ready to go home.

One particularly lonely day, Mary wandered into a church. She sat down in a pew and listened to people praying in French in a low voices. There was a rhythm to the prayer that reminded her of the prayers she'd said as a child. Calmness flooded over her. The familiar soothing tones and the connection with her childhood seemed to be just what she needed to recenter herself. Throughout the rest of her visit abroad she was able to stop self-soothing with food. She did this by recognizing when she was lonely or homesick, and then reciting one of her childhood prayers, which never failed to soothe her.

You don't have to be a spiritual or religious person to feel moved by a prayer. Chanting a repetitive prayer is simply one form of meditation. People who are comfortable and familiar with prayer often report feeling a positive shift in their mood after reciting a prayer several times.

~self-soothing technique~
Finding Your Mindful Spirit

1. Choose a short prayer or saying that holds special meaning for you. It could be a verse from the Bible or another spiritual book. Make sure you pick something very short, no longer than a few lines. Also, it must be something that you can repeat from memory. This phrase should connect with you or move you in a soulful way. Here are some suggestions: the twenty-third psalm, St. Francis's prayer, Buddha's discourse on good will, and the Serenity Prayer used by 12-step groups all across the world.

2. Repeat the verse several times until your urge to eat lessens.

3. If you can't find a verse or saying you like, or if you are still looking for one, try this meditational prayer:

   Tranquility in front of me.

   Calmness beside me.

   Stillness around me.

   Compassion inside me.

9. virtual bliss

My job is extremely stressful. I am a legal assistant who interviews people after they have been arrested for various crimes. Sometimes the stories people tell me get me very upset. But I have to appear calm and professional, even when I want to cry. I used to stress eat everyday. How do I cope now? Sometimes it's by detaching from the situation. I hung a picture of a gorgeous sunflower field across from my interview chair. After someone tells me a distressing story, I look at that picture and take a few minutes to recenter myself. I envision myself walking right into the picture. It calms me down enough to release me from the grip of my emotions. If not, I'd be barreling through snacks stashed in my desk the moment the client left the room. —Kate

Imagine for a moment that you are lying on the beach. The sun is warming your body. You're starting to feel relaxed and happy. The dark blue ocean's waves are breaking quietly against the rocks. You listen to that sound.

It's likely that a vivid, soothing image popped into your mind while you were reading the description above. This is a brief example of guided imagery. When you engage in *guided imagery*, you are actively directing your thoughts to a positive image. You mindfully guide your thoughts to a place where you feel soothed and comforted.

Guided imagery has been clinically proven to be a helpful technique for reducing binge eating (Esplen et al. 1998). It works because your mind and your body are intricately connected. When you imagine the feelings and sensations your body would encounter in your visualization, your body responds as if they were really happening. Imagine for a moment biting into a juicy peach. If you vividly call this image to mind, you are likely to start salivating. So, let's return to the image of you lying on a beach. Although you might not consciously notice a shift in your mood when you visualize a safe and relaxing place, be assured that your body is likely to respond by relaxing.

Have you ever visualized yourself cozying up to a pint of ice cream or vegging out with some "goodies" in front of the TV? If you do this, you are unintentionally using guided imagery as a way to increase stress eating rather than stop it. If you catch yourself unconsciously focusing on images that reinforce eating to self-soothe, don't be too hard on yourself. Just gently acknowledge this may set you up for mindless emotional eating. If you are stuck with this image, keep the guided imagery going, but this time change the ending. Instead, create an image of yourself successfully walking away from food and doing one of the nonfood alternative activities you'll find in this book.

~self-soothing technique~
Visualize a Soothing World Without Food

Guided imagery is a little like having a daydream. Use the power of your mind to paint a vivid picture of a safe, peaceful, and empowering atmosphere. It's a great alternative when you're a thousand miles away from an actual beach or you don't have enough cash for a spa. Visualization is a realistic option that can take the place of comfort foods.

- Mindfully create a new guided image. Choose a very peaceful place. It might be somewhere you once vacationed. It can also can be as simple as your actual bedroom or an imaginary garden. The important thing to remember is that it is a place where you feel safe and relaxed. When you think about this place, bring to mind all the sensory details. If it is at the ocean, think about the smells of the sea, the colors of the sky, and the temperature. If it is your bedroom, think about the texture of the pillow and the color of the comforter on your bed. It is important to bring as many sensory details to your mind as you can. This will stimulate different areas of your brain that can help you feel as if you are really there.

- Need some ideas? Try these: You can visualize drifting in a canoe on a quiet river, floating in outer space, strolling through an alpine meadow, hiking up a fire trail on a mountainside, soaking in a tub of hot water, sitting on a balcony overlooking the ocean, or lying on the warm sands of an island.

- If you are still having difficulty coming up with your own guided imagery, try focusing on a calming photograph. It could be a photo from a past vacation or a landscape painted by a famous painter.

- Practice replaying this scene many times in your head.

- If this doesn't work for you, there are many free audio guided imagery scenarios you can find on the Web.

10. ending hide-and-seek feelings

A food coma is what I call it. I slip into it when I overeat. Eating is like an emotional anesthetic. It takes me to a place where I don't feel anything. For example, I started eating a few days ago because I couldn't stand being so disappointed and angry at my boyfriend. I ate and then I ate some more. I didn't want to feel as bad as I was feeling. I also didn't want to accept the truth that he is not a very nice guy. If I had been brave enough to face the truth, I would have broken up with him immediately. Instead, I gained three pounds and I'm even more miserable. —Mary Ann

What is really at the core of emotional eating? Eating to get rid of uncomfortable emotions implies that there's something unacceptable about what you're feeling. You don't want to feel lousy, and you think that you can't stand feeling lousy for very long. Eating is one way to escape from your feelings by temporarily diverting your attention away from them (Heatherton and Baumeister 1991). You can't blame yourself for turning to something that works so well at providing you with temporary relief from negative feelings or general discomfort. But what if you had a higher tolerance for feeling bad?

Instead of trying to knock out your bad feelings with food, it might be possible for you to accept feeling bad and be able to live with that feeling for a while. It's normal to feel anger, disappointment, and stress sometimes. Learning to live with your negative emotions, instead of anesthetizing yourself from them with food, is called radical acceptance. *Radical acceptance* is, basically, a way of totally and completely focusing on what is, rather than what you want things to be. It is accepting the entire situation without trying to change it or fight against it. It's also an ancient technique for dealing with troubling emotions.

Emotional eating is the opposite of acceptance in many ways. It involves warding off feeling bad with comfort eating because you don't accept that this is the way you do feel. Acceptance doesn't mean you agree with or condone the situation. For example, when you are stressed-out, you probably don't like how you feel. Nor do you judge it to be a good thing. Nevertheless, it is the reality. When you stop fighting against how you are truly feeling, you'll find more productive ways to manage difficult emotions. You'll make a plan rather than stewing about how unfair it is that you feel that way. Getting to a place of radical acceptance isn't easy. But it is well worth your time to practice getting there.

~self-soothing technique~
Emotional Eating Acceptance Statements

When you feel the urge to emotionally eat, repeat the following acceptance statements to yourself. If you like, you can also make up your own acceptance statements:

- I radically accept myself.

- I accept my roller-coaster emotions with all of their ups and downs.

- I accept that I am tempted to use food to soothe myself.

- I accept that I am not perfect and will sometimes slip.

- I accept that I can feel this pain without numbing out with food.

- I accept that I cannot change how I feel.

- I surrender to this feeling and will commit to finding comfort in healthy ways that do not harm me.

~self-soothing technique~
Worst-Case Scenario

Here's a quick writing exercise to get to the bottom of those emotions that are so uncomfortable that you typically turn to food to feel better:

1. Ask yourself, what is so terrible about feeling the way that you do?

2. Is it likely that this amount of pain or discomfort will physically harm or kill you?

3. Does this feeling give you any important information? For example, overeating may be a sign that you are angrier than you realized.

4 change your thoughts, change your eating

If you want to change your emotional eating habits, you'll need to find ways to adapt how you think about the comforting properties of food. If you think only food can make you feel better in times of stress, you'll have a difficult time finding other ways to brighten your mood. It may take a lot of hard work to break your mental link between food and comfort, because it is such an ingrained notion. You also may benefit from putting a positive spin on your negative thoughts. Pessimistic thoughts only make you feel worse and may actually prompt your need for comfort. Your task in this chapter is to learn how to generate more soothing thoughts than the negative ones you may usually have. When you fill your mind with comforting and relaxing images and ideas, you lower the odds that you'll turn to food to deal with stress or negativity.

11. journaling to boost your mental health immunity

I'm clueless when it comes to my emotions. Journaling helps me understand my true motives for stress eating. When I write about my struggles, I often discover that I overeat because I am anxious about something. Eating calms my nerves. As I write, I don't judge myself. I just try to understand why I fell hook, line, and sinker for emotional eating again. I find clues for how I can be better prepared next time. —Olivia

Writing about your troubles is an easy and clinically proven way to help you soothe yourself (Keeling and Bermudez 2006). In fact, there is an entire branch of psychology devoted to the healing power of journaling. It's called *narrative therapy*. The theory is based on reauthoring (rewriting) and externalizing your feelings. Essentially, this means taking any feelings trapped inside you and describing them on paper so you can see them from another perspective. Unexamined feelings are like a strong undertow in the ocean. They can pull you in directions you may not want to go.

Why is journaling helpful? Well, it has several benefits. For starters, you are likely to have some aha experiences. Writing helps you be mindful of what drives you to eat for comfort. Many emotional eaters believe they eat just for the pleasure of eating, but often there is much more to it than that. Journaling helps you to confront the issue directly by examining it in depth. This contrasts with eating that numbs you and may cause you to avoid analyzing your feelings. After writing a journal entry, you may still want to eat for emotional reasons. But you will have a better understanding of why you feel that need in that moment.

The second benefit of journaling is that it can help you to think about your situation in a more positive, realistic way. Let's say Bob is having a bad day. He might tell himself, "This is the worst emotional eating I've ever done." But when he writes a journal entry, he realizes his recent bout of emotional eating was not the worst overeating he's ever done. It wasn't the amount of food that bothered him but the guilt and disappointment in himself. It was hard for him to see this until he put it down on paper.

Finally, journaling gives you an arena in which to plan for the next time you encounter the urge to stress eat. When you clearly spell out what your challenges were in the past, you can predict how you'll respond in the future, and you can make plans to deal with these challenges in a more productive way the next time.

Journaling 101: Writing Tips

- To make writing into a habit, plan to do it like clockwork at the same time each day. For example, you could take twenty minutes every morning before you have breakfast. Or you could write after you put the kids to bed at night.

- If you aren't into writing at length or you feel that you don't have the time, start by jotting down one or two notes in a day planner every day.

- Write without editing. Try not to censor yourself or erase. Just go with the flow. In psychology, this is called *free association*, which means allowing your mind to take you wherever it wants to go.

- For each journal entry, do a past, present, and future summary. The format is this: In the past, I felt about this issue... In the moment, I feel about this issue... And in the future, what would I like to do or say about this issue is...

- If you spend a great deal of time in front of a computer, try out a Web journal. There are many free online journaling services.

~self-soothing technique~
Investigating Stress Eating

If you are not sure what to write about, that's okay. There are some prompts below to help you get started. Each prompt is the beginning of a sentence. They are intended to stimulate your ideas. However, you don't need specific prompts to reap the benefits of writing. If the questions listed don't target what you're feeling, just pick up a pen or pencil and start writing.

- The worst thing about this situation is...

- Three adjectives that best describe how I feel in this moment are...

- The reason I'm feeling this emotion is…

- When I eat, I feel….

~self-soothing technique~
Looking at the Bright Side

Looking at the bright side can help you get out of a funk. It can also interrupt stress eating. After you read the following statements, take a fresh sheet of paper or open a new computer file to write about anything that comes to your mind. Chose only one statement and then write about it in as much detail as possible.

- A positive moment in your life, like your baby's first smile, a good report card, a job promotion, or a surprise birthday party

- A moment when you felt at peace or felt an intense calmness, like while you were watching a sunset on the shore of an ocean

- A moment when you fell in love

- A time you felt completely relaxed, such as on a vacation or a quiet moment after you put your children to bed

- A time when your sense of adventure was strong, such as a time you went somewhere you'd never gone to before or a time you tried something new, like scuba diving

Applying the Wisdom

When you have finished writing about any of the statements above, it's time to apply the wisdom. Answering the following questions may give you ideas on how to recreate some

Aspects of the positive moments in your life:

- What would it take to recreate such good feelings? How can you access even a bit of this emotion in the future?

- More specifically, how can those good feelings help you cope with emotional eating at a later date?

For example, say you wrote about a time when you felt completely relaxed on a vacation at the beach. You could write about any behaviors that would help you recreate some of the sensations from that experience. For instance, you could take your shoes off, put your bare feet into the bathtub, and run warm water over them. Then close your eyes and imagine walking along the water's edge at the beach. Perhaps you could play tropical music or call the friend who went with you to the beach to reminisce.

~self-soothing technique~
Image Journaling

No one ever said journals must be written. As the saying goes, A picture is worth a thousand words. Draw visual images of how you're feeling or take photographs of yourself in different moods. Keep a notebook of these drawings and photos. Date each picture and explain how it relates to food and emotional eating.

12. ha-ha moments

A good laugh is sometimes the best tranquilizer. The other day, I was down and depressed about my weight. I wanted to gorge myself on whatever I could find in the kitchen. Instead, I tried to relax on the couch. When I flipped on the TV, I saw an ancient episode of I Love Lucy. It was so silly that I rolled on the floor laughing. By the end of the episode, I had completely forgotten about food. My irritation had evaporated and I was able to get moving again. —Terri

Terri, a forty-two-year-old accountant, was once in a near-fatal airplane accident. While on her way to Europe, the plane had depressurized thousands of miles above the ocean. When the air masks were released, she was shaking so badly that she was unable to put on the mask. A nearby passenger came to her rescue. The plane made a safe emergency landing, but it was the most traumatic and terrifying situation in Terri's entire life. In therapy ten days after the safe landing, she was still trembling. She became tearful when she recounted the details. Since the event, she had lost control of her eating.

Two years later, Terri tells the same story in a very different way. She laughs as she demonstrates how her hands trembled when she tried to put the air mask over her face. Getting in touch with her laughter took some time. Initially, laughter was a physical release that was better than crying. Then when she retold how the event had happened, she noticed that laughing helped her and others to be less traumatized by the details. Friends were able to give her support instead of becoming overwhelmed by the story. The experience also demonstrated to Terri how comical it can be to stress about trivial matters when much worse things can happen.

This incident is, of course, an extreme example. Most stressful events that prompt overeating aren't so terrifying. It's interesting that an experience can be so terrible in the moment, but later on you can see the humor in the situation. Humor is an extremely powerful therapeutic tool. It is a recognized way of coping with some hurts, and it can be amazingly healing (Thorson et al. 1997; Tugade, Fredrickson, and Barrett 2004). Laughter boosts the immune system and decreases stress hormones. It's also linked to lowering blood pressure, which can be a key factor in stress management. The chemical changes produced by laughter are very much like the mood-elevating benefits of exercise.

If you experience debilitating guilt or shame for mindless emotional eating, laughter is a great way to redirect your focus away from feeling bad, and it can brighten your mood, as well.

~self-soothing technique~
Laughing Yoga

Laughing yoga is a modern new form of yoga. It was created by a family physician in Mumbai, India, and the practice has spread worldwide since its invention. The idea behind laughing yoga (*hasya yoga*) or any kind of humor therapy is that laughter is another way to change the sensations in the body. When you start laughing, the physical movements create a cascade of reactions in your body. Your brain sends signals to your body to relax, while at the same time, particular neurotransmitters are released that help you feel pleasure. Laughing exercises relieve tension and distract you from negative feelings. They also provide a workout for your abs, diaphragm, and shoulders while you are making the natural movements associated with laughter.

Jump right in and give it a try. Repeat these laughter sounds out loud in a jolly Santa Claus manner: Ho ho. Ha ha ha. Repeat them several times for a few minutes. It's likely that your simulated laughter will turn into real laughter. Playacting your way from fake laughter is a great way to help you arrive at true laughter. Think of it as being like the canned laughter on TV sitcoms. Did you ever notice that just hearing the canned laughter sometimes made you join in? You can also check out videos on the Web for examples of how to do laughing yoga.

~self-soothing technique~
Medicinal Laughter

- Find the natural humor in whatever problem you're struggling with. To help, look to the future. What about this situation might cause you to laugh five years from today? Is there anything giggle worthy in it? For example, is there a Three Stooges moment? Try to imagine how your favorite comedian would take this situation and turn it into a humorous sketch.

- Do something funny. Leave a funny phone message for a friend. Make up a fictional name and use it all day. Wear a T-shirt or a hat that makes people laugh.

- Learn a one-line joke and tell it to everyone you meet in your day.

- Put a funny picture of yourself or an amusing picture from a magazine on your refrigerator door. You can even tape the picture onto a box of cookies in your cupboard so that when you start searching for food to snack on, you'll see it.

Some situations are just not funny and humor is not appropriate. If your problem really doesn't have any comic elements, try to find humor elsewhere. Take your mind off your problem by going to funny websites or renting a funny movie. No matter what prompts your laughter, it will do good things for your body and mind.

13. when you feel empty, choose feeling that your glass is half full

I messed up again! Chocolate chip cookies sent all my good efforts to eat well back to square one. Why can't I get anything right? I feel I'm a complete failure. How hard is it to control myself? I allow myself a little pity party before remembering that I'm working on looking at the bright side. I must remember that this isn't a make-or-break situation, even thought it feels like one. The good news is that there are no more cookies in the house. At least that temptation is gone and I can start again—right now. As my mother used to say, "You have to break some eggs to make an omelet." —Kathy

Therapists are experts at helping people feel better. When you consider that they have only words to comfort their clients, it's amazing. No hugs. No gifts. No food. This is intriguing. They must use very powerful words and string them together very skillfully to get the results they do. So what is their secret? Partly, it's that they give people support and encouragement. But what exactly do they say that helps people feel better even in their worst moments?

Much of what therapists do is to *reframe* the situation. The therapist explains how the client feels from another perspective than the one the client has. Instead of focusing on the problem a particular issue creates for you, reframing looks at the benefits or opportunities presented by that difficult issue.

Let me describe a common situation that many stress eaters face. Emotional eaters focus a lot on their failures. They have laundry lists of everything they've done wrong and condemn themselves for falling back into old habits. Here is one way to reframe this particular situation: those overeating moments aren't really failures. Instead, they're *missteps*. These missteps provide you with useful information to study and use to guide you. They are teaching moments that help you identify what you need to work on. The good news is that you can do such reframing yourself. You don't need a Ph.D. in psychology to get a new perspective on your situation. You just have to look at it differently. As the saying goes, When life gives you lemons, make lemonade. When you reframe a situation, you take charge of how you think about the issue.

~self-soothing technique~
Practice the Art of Reframing

1. Evaluate your language. Write down any negative words that you use to describe the situation (failure, stupid, worst ever, and so forth).

2. Choose new words. For example, change "failure" to "stumble." A "relapse" can be made into a "reminder" or even a "chance to start again."

3. Consider how you can use this experience as a teaching moment. A *teaching moment* means taking a difficult situation and weaving an important lesson into

it. We often see teaching moments with kids. If your toddler makes a negative remark about someone's weight, that's a good moment to talk to the child about being sensitive to others and accepting them, no matter what they look like.

4. Now get a pen or pencil and a stack of 3 by 5 index cards. Write down a valuable lesson that you learned from a particular situation you are currently dealing with or from an earlier experience. Post this card in an easy-to-see location.

Let's say you just had an episode of emotional eating. And let's say that you tried to use a breathing technique to stop mindlessly snacking in the kitchen, but it didn't work. You could reframe this incident as "good information." Why? Perhaps this incident taught you that if you first get yourself out of the kitchen, the breathing exercise might work better. Write this advice on the 3 by 5 card.

You can use reframes in two ways: They can help you change your perception of a stressful situation. Or you can use them to help you cope and recover from incidents of comfort eating. Let's say you ate a bag of M&M's when you weren't really hungry, and now you feel guilty. You can say the following statements to yourself, not to condone emotional eating, but to encourage you to move forward:

- This is a challenge, not a problem.

- With crisis comes opportunity.

- This is a learning experience. It is a great lesson.

- Someday I will laugh about it, and it will be a great story to tell.

- This could be much worse. I have it better than some others do.

- It's great just to be alive. Hurt is a part of life.

- The glass is half full, not half empty.

- There are more things I like about myself than the one thing I focus on disliking.

- Stressing-out is a waste of time. Everything will come out alright.

- Everything happens for a reason. I have faith in that.

14. daydreaming the blues away

I used to find myself daydreaming about food. I'd drift off into a land that's a little like Willy Wonka's chocolate factory. Now I have a variety of recurring, comforting daydreams to choose from. One is a about a vacation on the beach. Another is about cuddling with my boyfriend on a stormy night with a glass of wine. The last one is about winning the lottery. (I can dream can't I?) I take a long time thinking about all the things I would do with the money. Daydreaming about happy things distracts me from food fantasies and comforts me. —Wendy

Wendy hates feeling out of control. Any situation that seems completely out of her hands feels awful. She used to find herself fantasizing about food when she felt so upset and out of control. Now she turns to her mind to steady herself. In her personal fantasyland, she has complete control over where her mind travels and what she is feeling, even if she doesn't have that kind of control in real life. Feeling mentally in charge is very soothing to Wendy and it is a nice option when what she really wants to comfort herself is not available. For example, Wendy often dreams about being pampered in a spa, even if there is no spa in her immediate environment. There's no doubt that daydreaming can fill the time that you might be thinking about food with other things that are pleasurable to think about. It also helps to curb the eating Wendy does when she is bored. Fantasizing about going on a vacation or buying a new outfit can distract and soothe Wendy for quite a long time.

Try to steer clear of imagining yourself eating in your daydreams. Sometimes people daydream about what they're going to eat for dinner, luscious desserts, or even what would taste great right in the moment. Most likely this will only increase food cravings. If you find yourself daydreaming about food, stop and actively redirect your thoughts to a more neutral or positive fantasy, such as going on a desired vacation or being with someone you love.

~self-soothing technique~
Soothing Aspirations

Create a poster with a visual array of pleasurable activities. Use images that relate to your daydreams and to healthy ways to soothe yourself. Making a poster like this is not a new concept. Goal charts and vision boards have been around for a long time. This task is unique, however, because it is not focused on material things or goals for success. Instead, you will create a visual image to remind yourself that there are many ways to soothe yourself that do not involve eating or food.

This exercise activates your visual memory. Some people are very strong visual learners. They need to see something to remember it, instead of reading or hearing about it. Looking at a picture is another route for encoding memory. When you're seeking ways to calm down, an image from this poster might pop into your mind.

1. Buy a piece of heavy poster board (8½ by 11 inches or 11 by 14 inches).

2. Get a stack of magazines. It would be helpful to have several different genres represented, like health, nature, news, and women's magazines.

3. Close your eyes and think for a moment. Or look through the magazines for inspiration. Ask yourself, "What do I find soothing besides food?" Cut out pictures of someone meditating or doing yoga. Find a picture of a sunset or someone sailing on a placid lake. When you are feeling the urge to stress eat, these images will represent the type of calmness you'd like to have. Paste them down on the board.

4. You can also add words of encouragement or even poems to the images on the board. Include motivational words, phrases, and affirmations.

5. Include images of fun activities and places you daydream about visiting.

6. There is one rule: stay away from unhealthy images, even if they're enticing. That means no skinny supermodels. Don't use pictures of overweight people either. (Some people try to scare themselves away from overeating.) When you look at this picture, remember that you want to create a soothing effect, not a frightening one.

7. Display your poster where you'll see it frequently; for example, above your desk, on your bathroom door, or somewhere in your kitchen.

15. worry mindfully

I seem to worry about twenty times a day. Mostly I worry about my fiancé. He hates his boss. They don't treat him fairly at work. Every night I make dinner for the two of us. Then I pick at the meal as I anxiously wait for him to come home. I find myself worrying about how things went at work for him that day, and what kind of mood he will be in when he walks in the door. —Lori

We all worry way too much. Many of us spend too many of our waking hours obsessing about things we can't control, and we become distraught about situations that may or may not occur. Although we know it isn't good for us, it's very hard to stop. "Worry eaters" is the term used for people who nibble or graze on food as a way to cope with their fretting. They are often drawn to eating because it feels as though they are doing something besides worrying. However, whatever you are worrying about is often out of your control. Most of the time, there is nothing you can do to change the outcome of the situation. As a result, you may feel a strong urge to get busy. Unfortunately, cooking and snacking give you something to do.

If you are in the habit of eating when you worry, it might help to do something that feels productive. Ask yourself what you have the power to do in the moment. Then focus on creating a plan to make it happen. For example, if you are worried about your finances, make a budget. Take charge of what you can control. It will feel very good.

A major downside to worrying is that it uses a lot of time and emotional energy. It also jeopardizes your health and may cause you to lose sleep or feel physically ill. For emotional eaters, worry definitely can increase your vulnerability to overeating. When distracted by concerns, you're less invested in what you put into your mouth. You can eat when your mind is elsewhere, particularly when you're caught in a whirlwind of worry.

Also, worry is often the result of overeating rather than the cause. You can find yourself fretting about how much you just ate. But in that situation, you can't control or change what happened. Focus on what you can do, now that the act of eating is over. Worrying about weight gain won't make you feel better. Taking a walk will.

~self-soothing technique~
Worry Mindfully

One way to avoid nervous snacking is to worry mindfully. When you usually worry, it's likely that your attention is divided between what you're doing (or munching on) and the issue you're worrying about. Instead of dividing your attention that way, carve out some time from your day to give your worry your full attention.

Here's an example: When your mind begins to fret about something, say to yourself, "Not yet, I'll get back to this later." Postpone worrying until later that evening. Then, when you've got the time, give yourself a good twenty minutes to worry. Set a timer so you won't have to be concerned about the time. During the period you devote to this task, remember not to do anything else. Ask yourself, "What is the worst-case scenario for what I'm worrying about?" For a moment, visualize what would happen in this worst-case scenario. When you do this, you often find that your image isn't a realistic fear or that it's something that you wouldn't like but could survive.

~self-soothing technique~
Worry Beads

Get a set of *komboloi*, which is the Greek word for worry beads. Traditionally, komboloi are used to help people relieve their worries when they're fidgety or need to pass the time. The beads are popular because they're believed to provide an antidote to a variety of unhealthy habits, such as biting your nails, overeating, smoking, and worrying. They work because massaging the beads with your hands has a calming and soothing effect. If you can't find these worry beads, make your own. You can put as many beads on a string as you like. Cut a piece of yarn or string as long as the palm of your hand. Then tie a knot on one end and slide some beads onto the string. Tie a knot on the other end, leaving some slack between the beads so your thumb can release one bead to the next finger. The cord should provide enough space for the beads to move easily. Listen to the sounds the beads make as they fall from one end of the cord to the other. You can click the beads in any rhythm that you find calming.

16. zone out mindfully

When I get home from work, I am psychologically exhausted. I can't handle one more question or chore. I make a beeline for an after-work snack. I need a bite to eat but I end up eating enough for a meal. Eating keeps my hands busy while I slip into an alternate dimension where I can't think. I don't really know what I am doing. I completely zone out like a zombie while I mechanically munch on snacks. When I'm done, it's like I'm suddenly jolted out of a food coma. I think, "Oh, what have I done?" —Jennifer

Jennifer comes home from work, stares blankly at the TV, and munches mindlessly on food for an hour. Like many people, Jennifer eats simply to zone out from the world for a while. This trancelike state shuts down her thoughts and dulls the sensations in her body. For Jennifer, this is a welcome change for her overloaded mind. Unfortunately, zoned-out snacking is a mental break that can be dangerously enticing.

There are many ways to experience zoning out, or resting your brain. Maybe you've tuned out during a conversation, or even spaced out while driving a car. When you wake up from mental cruise control, you realize that you've passed your destination and become aware of how mentally detached you were from driving. It's pretty scary that you can drive, talk, and eat normally for a short while with very little thought involved. Eating to zone out can be drastically reduced when you have alternative ways to relax your brain. It all begins with giving yourself permission to shut down your mind, which may be a foreign concept if you multitask and juggle many different tasks at once.

~self-soothing technique~
Blank Mind

If you use food as a way to zone out, try out alternative ways to get a short mental break. Focus on repetitive, monotonous tasks. But first, get into the right frame of mind. Sit down. Give yourself permission to zone out. This part can be hard for busy moms, for type A personalities, or if you just have trouble sitting still. To help you work on emptying your mind, first imagine dumping out the contents of a wastepaper basket. Then imagine all the thoughts in your brain are pouring out of your head in the same way that you emptied the wastepaper basket. Now pick a mindless activity to do:

- Try flipping through a magazine. This is an activity that is barely active, mildly amusing, and doesn't require any mental effort at all. Reading a book takes too much mental energy. But just looking at pictures and scanning through photos is enough to decompress mindlessly and can also absorb nervous energy.

- Watch TV. Turning on the TV can often help you zone out. Sometimes, however, it just isn't active enough to keep you distracted. If watching TV doesn't do it for you, try flipping the channels. Make sure you aren't with others, as this will drive them a little crazy. This is similar to flipping through a magazine. The many images flashing before your eyes stimulate your mind and senses but don't require any active mental work.

- Do you want to zone out totally? Try closing your eyes. Focus on staring at the void and the blackness on the inside of your eyelids.

- Get back to basics. Think about some of the things you liked to do as a child. There is nothing more calming than nostalgic memories from childhood, like shaping Play-Doh or coloring mindlessly. Playing doesn't use much mental energy, and it's fun, stimulates your imagination, and boosts your energy.

- Try origami, the ancient Japanese art of folding paper. Go to origami.com for hundreds of examples. This is a very easy and mindless activity that will keep your hands busy and out of the cookie jar.

17. the Scarlett O'Hara approach

How do I sabotage my diet? I have a hundred different ways. But the one that gets me into the most trouble is when I use food to stall. If I want to procrastinate, I suddenly feel that I really need a snack. I can waste a lot of time poking around the kitchen getting a snack. —Ellen

"I can't think about that now. I'll think about it tomorrow." These are the famous words of Scarlet O'Hara from the classic novel *Gone with the Wind*. She was actually juggling quite a bit of stress: being caught in the middle of a war-torn country, losing (she thought) the love of her life to another woman, and marrying men she didn't love for financial stability. It was a lot for a girl to handle. So what did she do? She decided that she couldn't worry about some of it right then. Mentally, Scarlett put her worries on an imaginary shelf, and she took them out only when she was ready to handle them.

Shelving a problem is different from avoiding or ignoring it. *Shelving* a problem means to approach the issue strategically and commit to dealing with it at a specific time. As the saying has it, Timing is everything. This idea is quite like putting away the pictures of your ex after a difficult breakup. When you're upset, pictures can trigger mournful thoughts and keep you stuck in dwelling on the breakup. When you're ready to see them without becoming depressed, you can look at them again.

Shoebox It

Snacking is often an avoidance technique. If you allow yourself to tackle a problem when you are truly ready instead of rushing into it, you may not have to find ways to stall. And you may not have to keep yourself so busy with food that you won't have time to deal with the problem. Reassure yourself that it's okay to hold on to some of your problems and that when you're ready, you'll deal with them mindfully.

To use this technique, you'll create a box that will be the temporary storage place for anything bothering you that you can't deal with at this moment. You can use a ready-made box or you can make your own. When you struggle with a problem, write about it. Then stuff the piece of paper into the box. If you aren't near your box, imagine putting your problem into the box. Where can you put your box until you're ready to deal with the problem? The top shelf of your closet? Under your bed? In a drawer? When you feel ready to deal with the problem, get the box and open it. Commit to taking just one step at a time to deal with this difficult issue. Write a list of the needed steps. Then deal with only one task at a time.

18. finding your security blanket

I carry around a special pen in my pocket. I got it the day I graduated from college. I have a learning disability. Graduating was the proudest moment of my entire life. Whenever I get upset, I hold on to the pen. It comes out during stressful meetings and conflicts with my landlord. I grip it tightly. No one really notices. Lately, the pen helps me cope with the urge to emotionally overeat. Sometimes I hold it just to remind me what it feels like to be proud of myself. I feel very good about myself when I don't use eating to feel good. If I'm angry and want to stress eat, I scribble on a piece of paper. If I get into boredom eating, I doodle with my pen until the craving for food has thankfully passed. Sometimes I even chew on it. —Morgan

Linus from Charles M. Shultz's Peanuts cartoon was very attached to his security blanket. As most little kids do, he took it everywhere. You could see why he'd need something to make him feel better. Lucy, his sister, and Sally, his friend, were constantly tormenting him. Although you have likely grown out of your need for a security blanket, we all take comfort from objects that hold special meaning for us.

These objects are what psychologists call transitional objects. A *transitional object* is a physical object that replaces the mother-child bond and allows for the development of a separate self, much like the way Linus uses his blanket. A blanket or teddy bear is a substitute for the cozy comfort of a mother. As a toddler, the child may move on to an imaginary friend or special stuffed animal. As we get older, we may treasure sentimental items that have no value other than how we feel about them, such as a particular picture, a coffee mug, or a pillow. It can lift your mood when you look at it.

It's likely that you own a transitional object. It might be a lucky rabbit's foot or a shell your lover picked up during a romantic stroll on the beach. Sometimes you may carry it around in your pocket to touch, or you may find that rubbing it can shift you into a better mood. If you have such an object, it may be helpful to keep it close by. You never know when you may be tempted to snack your way to a better mood, and this object might help you not do that.

~self-soothing technique~
Finding a Soothing Object

- Spend some time identifying items around your home that hold sentimental meaning for you. You might find an article of clothing. Or it could be a card someone sent you for your birthday. Place these items in a special box. Put the box aside so the items in it are ready when you need them. Do this task well before you are in need of those items.

- Note that this book can be a transitional object for you. When you need comfort, just pick it up and flip through the pages. Reading various passages aloud or just holding it might make you feel better. You may feel comforted and understood.

• Jewelry can be an especially good soothing item. It doesn't have to be expensive. It just has to be special to you in some way. Maybe it was given to you by your soul mate. Perhaps your great-aunt gave you a necklace before she died because you were her favorite. Maybe you bought a bracelet as a special gift to yourself for getting a promotion. Bracelets, necklaces, and rings are great because you can wear them all the time and touch them when you need a moment of comfort. Be careful not to choose jewelry that saddens you, like a ring from your ex-husband. If you don't have any jewelry, that's okay. Look around your home for other objects with sentimental value. Slip a ticket stub from your favorite band into your purse or put a photo that always makes you smile into your wallet. If you can find something that fits into your hand or pocket, that's very helpful.

19. soothing affirmations

*I read that affirmations can help me to be more positive. I'm
a bit of a pessimist. When something could or does go wrong,
I stress out and then eat myself silly. So I wrote three positive
statements and pasted them on the refrigerator. I committed to
saying each one out loud at least once a day. What did I have to
lose? At first, I felt really dumb. But I kept doing it anyway. I
know the exact moment it clicked. I was having a hard day and
was about to open a candy bar when I heard myself say inside my
head, "It's not the end of the world. Tomorrow will be better."
I put down the candy bar. This was an affirmation I had on
the refrigerator! It had popped into my mind with no effort at
all. Somehow it had crept into my subconscious when I wasn't
looking. It's a pretty painless way to lighten up and stop pigging
out on food when I'm stressed-out.* —Brenda

Buddha said, "What you think, you become." Although this
statement is centuries old, it still holds true. If you think posi-
tively, you will act in more uplifting ways. If you think you can
calm yourself down without food, you will act in ways that will
help you to do exactly that. If you don't think it's possible, you
won't even try. For this reason, your thoughts hold an enormous
amount of power.

So how can you convince yourself that soothing yourself
without food is possible after so many years of doing the opposite? Affirmations are a helpful step. Affirmations are positive,
affirming statements about yourself. They're the opposite of negative self-talk. You can use affirmations to retrain your brain to

think confidently and optimistically about your ability to choose nonfood methods to calm yourself down.

Critical self-talk can hold you back and damage your confidence that you can change your unhealthy food habits. Affirmations focus your mind on positive thoughts and help you hold on to the idea that change is possible (Epton and Harris 2008). Also, you can direct affirmations toward many different aspects of your life. Here are some to use for specific purposes:

- *Physical:* I have a healthy body.

- *Emotional:* I am a strong person and a survivor. I've coped with many difficult things in my life. I can cope with emotional eating too.

- *Intellectual:* I'm a smart person. I can find many logical ways to soothe myself that will work better than eating.

- *Creative:* I know how to think outside of the box. I can find many solutions to stress eating.

- *Relationships:* I deserve respect. When I take care of my body, I am respecting myself.

~self-soothing technique~
Encouraging Words to End Stress Eating

Adopting a more positive outlook takes some effort and practice. Say the following statements out loud several times a day.

You can train your mind to bring affirming statements into your consciousness automatically. Choose one or more that resonate with you. Write the statements on cards and place them in easy-to-see locations, like your car's dashboard, a mirror, a door, or on your telephone.

When you say these affirmations, try to stay in the present. Instead of saying, "I will learn how to stop stress eating," say, "I am learning how to stop stress eating right now." Here are some examples you may find helpful:

- I'm on the road to feeling calmer.

- Eating won't resolve this problem.

- I'm good at tackling a challenge head-on.

- I can do this. It just takes time.

- I can wait. My hunger will pass with a little patience.

- I can soothe myself. I don't need food to do that.

- I am going to feel less stressed any minute. I can hang in here.

- I enjoy being healthy.

- I feel good inside, and my outer body is just about to catch up with me.

20. from Ms. Perfectionist to Ms. Realistic

There is nothing more maddening than me telling myself, "Well, you blew it, so you might as well give in completely." These words take away any chance I have of stopping the stress eating before it's too late. —Terri

Terri struggles with what some of my clients have creatively named "zebra thinking," or what is more traditionally thought of as black-and-white thinking. *Zebra thoughts* are extreme statements with little flexibility or room for shades of gray. "I always screw up," is a good example of zebra thinking. Most likely the word "always" isn't completely true. Words like "always" and "never" overstate the facts. Nonzebra thinking is less extreme and often more accurately describes the situation. For example, it's probably true that you engage in stress eating sometimes, rather than always. The more polarized you become in your thinking, the more extreme your reaction may be.

Emotional eaters tend to be very good at zebra thinking. They feel that they either must eat just right or else all of their eating is completely wrong. This way of thinking frequently happens automatically, and sometimes it isn't in the emotional eater's awareness. It's important to be aware of your own zebra thinking. This mind-set can talk you into overeating or into giving up completely. Zebra thinking doesn't see the difference between a little emotional eating and a lot. And there is a big difference!

Letting Go of Zebra Thinking

Your task is to break out of old ways of black-and-white think-ing. Here are some tips for actively choosing more soothing and realistic thoughts.

- **Watch for trigger words.** This includes absolute terms like "always," "never," "ever," "perfect," "disaster," and "impossible." If you hear yourself saying these words, try to counter them with a less extreme term, like "sometimes," "occasionally," "good enough" and so on. In the context of eating, typically these words form sentences like "I'm a complete failure," "I've totally ruined everything," and "I will never be able to stop stress eating." Instead, focus on a more realistic statement, such as "I am often able to soothe myself with activities other than eating."

- **Set up realistic expectations.** Feeling overwhelmed is often partly due to unrealistic goals that you can't possibly achieve. Emotional eaters are notorious for setting themselves up for failure. Statements like "I will eat only healthy foods tomorrow," or "I will never eat another donut" are zebra statements. You have to give yourself some leeway that you might slip up here and there.

- **The two-minute rule.** Emotional eaters often feel that they must do things perfectly or they give up. They think they'll do half an hour of exercise or none at all. Instead, whatever it is, commit to trying it out for just two minutes. For example, try just two minutes of a self-soothing technique. See what happens.

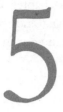 soothing
sensations to
calm and relax
the body

Much of stress eating is really about finding a way to unwind and relax. Chewing a hamburger or licking an ice cream cone is relaxing and pleasurable to the body. The good news is that there are a number of healthy ways to soothe your nerves and body that have nothing to do with eating. In this chapter, your task will be to try out new ways to relax. An increased awareness of your body helps you to take better care of yourself. Fortunately, your body is one of the best natural tools you have to cope with the rush and stressfulness of everyday life. There are lots of healthy ways to calm your body. In this chapter, you will learn about relaxation techniques, exercise, yoga, and ways to pamper your senses. Soothing your body can train your mind to become less reactive to stress.

stress and your body

Your body often takes the brunt of stress and stress eating. People who are chronically stressed often exhibit the evidence. They tend to catch more colds due to their lower immunity, and they get gray hair earlier in life. Feeling overwhelmed and over-burdened causes people to either lose or gain a lot of weight. Moreover, when you are living with chronic stress, your body holds on to weight by storing it in your belly region. The impact of stress on your body makes a strong case for finding healthy ways to soothe yourself rather than potentially harming yourself with emotional eating.

Let's take a brief look at what stress does to your body. In general, when you experience a threat or danger, the HPA axis (comprised of the hypothalamus, pituitary, and adrenal glands) becomes activated. It signals your body to release the stress hormones cortisol and adrenaline, as well as the neurotransmitter norepinephrine. These substances produce the fight-or-flight response that prepares your body to deal with a stressful event. This complex response affects your body in many ways. One way is the manner in which you crave food and store energy.

You may have noticed that your desire for sugary, fatty, and salty foods skyrockets when you are under a lot of pressure.

That's because your body tries to restore the balance of your hormones and neurotransmitters quickly and naturally. When the stress continues and your body is unable to return to its natural equilibrium, your body sends signals to your brain that it needs to find a way to restore balance. Often you do this by seeking foods that will regulate your neurotransmitters and stress hormones and temporarily boost your energy.

When you can calm down, you lessen the physiological and chemical stress reactions that are taking place. For this reason, how you cope with stress has a direct impact on your body. Your job is to quiet your mind and calm the physical response you have to stress. Soothing your body can help you return to equilibrium naturally after being flooded with stress hormones and, in turn, help regulate your appetite.

21. pampering your senses

Ahhh. This is the sound that escapes from my lips the moment I take a sip of hot tea. It stops me from emotional eating because I actually enjoy drinking it. I crave the warmth spreading throughout my body as I slowly sip. I try to let go of my worries and follow the sensation as my body warms up, just as if I were sitting next to a cozy fireplace. —Carmela

There really isn't any mystery about why some foods are so soothing. The scent of freshly baked cinnamon rolls smells like heaven to your nose. A bowl of hot beef stew warms up your body on a cold day. A dish of creamy ice cream can cool your tongue while it stimulates your taste buds for sweetness. People often seek the comfort of food because it is one way of pleasing their senses. Fortunately, there are a lot of healthy, noncaloric ways to improve your awareness of your sensations—that is, to improve the quality of what you see, hear, touch, taste, and smell.

~self-soothing technique~
Slipping into Soothing Sensations

When you are looking for comfort, try calming one or more of your senses. You'll be amazed at how well this lessens the need to emotionally eat.

- **Light therapy.** Sunlight or bright full-spectrum light on your skin can significantly improve your mood.

It's one of the main forms of treatment for seasonal affective disorder (SAD), which is a mild form of depression some people experience during the winter months when there is little sunlight (Golden et al. 2005). Sunlight helps reset your internal clock and increases your serotonin levels. When you feel you need comfort, sit by a window in indirect sunlight or go outdoors for thirty minutes—but don't forget to use sunscreen and sunglasses. If there's very little sunlight in the wintertime where you live or if you can't get outdoors, investigate buying a therapy light. These are bright lights you can use indoors that have the same healing effect as sunlight does.

- **Sip hot or cold tea.** If there's a pattern to your stress eating, you may want to schedule teatime for yourself at some point in the day when you might be prone to eat for emotional reasons. Tea is chemically complex. It has many different ingredients that affect neurotransmitters and other mood-regulating chemicals. Black tea has been shown to lower cortisol, a stress hormone (Steptoe et al. 2006). Chamomile is one type of herbal tea well-known for its soothing and calming properties.

- **Apply a warm or cold washcloth.** To calm your body, put a damp washcloth over your eyes, feet, or forehead. Choose a warm or cool cloth depending on what sounds the most soothing to you at the moment.

- **Wrap up in a blanket; cocoon yourself.** Not only will this warm you up, but pulling an afghan around your body can make you feel very protected and soothed. You might also want to invest in soft flannel sheets and a heavy comforter to cover yourself in bed.

- **Buy an inexpensive fountain.** The sound of water cascading is very relaxing and pleasant to the ears. In recent years, affordable small desktop waterfalls have become available.

- **Wear your favorite outfit.** Put on your favorite cozy sweater or the skirt that people always compliment. Wearing attractive clothing can be a great pick-me-up for days when you aren't feeling at your best.

22. soothing scents to rejuvenate yourself

The smell of warm cinnamon buns sends me from zero to crazy in ten seconds flat. Just one sniff of the aroma triggers all kinds of emotions. It's amazing how the scent, even if the cinnamon rolls aren't anywhere in sight, creates a frantic need to eat them. Other aromas are comforting to me. I love to light a jasmine-scented candle. I inhale slowly. The smell of lavender is also amazingly soothing. It isn't as yummy as a piece of pie. But a small whiff can create an instant Zen mood. —Melanie

The ability to smell is hardwired in the brain in a very different way than the ability to hear, see, taste, or touch. Scents are processed directly by the brain instead of being relayed through other brain structures, as with your other senses. Memories are often triggered by scents because they affect the *hippocampus*, the brain structure that stores memories. Smells also impact the *amygdala*, the brain organ that mediates emotions. This is why a whiff of freshly cut grass may bring back very powerful memories of being a kid playing outdoors. The smell is encoded in your brain along with your memories and emotions.

Versions of aromatherapy have been around for a very long time. The ancient Greeks and Romans relied on essential oils as perfumes. The original Olympic athletes rubbed scented oils into their muscles to soothe tension. Aromatic oils were well-known staples in ancient Eastern medicine. There are many references to the use of oils in the Bible. In recent years, these ancient practices of aromatherapy have been tested and found to have physical, emotional, and cognitive benefits (Moss et al. 2008).

In general, soothing scents have many positive effects. A pleasant aroma acts quickly to soothe you, much like food. Its effect is immediate. Pleasant aromas have no side effects, in contrast to drugs and antidepressants. It can't hurt to try some. Although catching a whiff of hot brownies can cause a lot of tension and make you afraid that you might overeat, many aromas don't have that effect. They don't generate any worries about weight gain.

~self-soothing technique~
Sensational Scents

If the scent of baking bread or sizzling bacon stimulates your appetite, try curbing it with changing the scent entering your nose as quickly as possible. Scents can be administered in two ways: absorbed through the skin or through olfactory channels.

Go to a health food store and investigate the essential oils. Look for 100 percent essential oils, which are the substances linked with soothing and calming tension. Stash some in your desk at work. Take a few whiffs when you're tempted to take an afternoon stroll to the vending machine. Or carry a bottle in your purse.

Don't know which scent to choose? The most soothing scent is said to be lavender. Other soothing scents are chamomile, rose, peppermint, lemon, eucalyptus, and lemongrass. But, keep in mind that what smells good to you is a matter of personal preference. Test a few scents and find one that works for you.

For the worried eater or night eater: Wash your sheets with a hint of lavender. Lie down on the lavender-scented sheet for a while when you need to decompress emotionally or when you are tempted to stress eat. The scent also may help you to sleep better at night.

For the grazer: If you find yourself grazing on food, light a scented tea candle. A tea candle is very small and generally burns quickly. Agree to delay eating until the tea candle burns out. It is likely that your craving for food will pass while you are waiting and focusing on the soothing scent.

For the anxious eater: You can combine scents with massage. Massage scented oil on your feet, wrists, or neck. If you want to smell the scent as well, try rubbing a little on your earlobe. Be careful about which scents you choose. Make sure to get a doctor's approval and to read the label. **Caution:** Some herbal scents applied directly to your skin can be absorbed into your bloodstream or may irritate your skin.

Eating from boredom and to unwind: Rosemary and jasmine are invigorating scents. For boredom eaters, stimulating your brain with energizing scents may be helpful. If you don't have any scents available, you may have to improvise. Coffee is a powerful aroma that many people find calming and stimulating at the same time. Keep a plastic bag of aromatic coffee beans in your purse. Be sure to close the bag tightly or your entire purse will become saturated with the scent.

23. yoga 101

Yoga is the only thing that works for me. I can't exercise because of my bad knees. But yoga poses are easy for me to do. After doing a few poses, I feel more relaxed. I'm not so dead set on stress eating. It loosens up the muscles that get tight from all the tension and stress I'm carrying. —Natalie

Natalie was like many emotional eaters. Initially, she turned her nose up at yoga, saying, "It doesn't make you sweat like aerobics. So how is it going to help me manage my weight?" Natalie soon changed her mind. Let me tell you why.

Yoga may not always make you sweat, but it can help you cope with the urge to nibble between meals. It can also curb stress eating (Boudette 2006; Daubenmier 2005). Basically, yoga teaches you how to have a strong mind-body connection. Strengthening this relationship allows you to listen to your body better. When you slow down and turn your attention to your stomach, you begin to know more accurately what it wants and needs.

Your body sends you cues that let you know when you are hungry and when you are full. But you have to be able to recognize them. Yoga teaches you how to tune in to your body's sensations so that you can feel your body and know it well. Then you can more accurately distinguish emotional hunger from physical hunger. When you are truly mentally present and in the moment, which you learn how to be in yoga, you are aware of your body's internal movements. This awareness prevents you from mindlessly popping food into your mouth when you are anxious or upset.

Natalie began practicing yoga every day. She soon noticed the benefits that many people who do yoga often describe. She increased her flexibility and stamina and strengthened her muscles. When she was tense, she did a few yoga poses to relax instead of munching on food, as she used to do. Cutting out stress eating from her life caused her to lose weight, even though she never sweated.

~self-soothing technique~
Strike a Yoga Pose

When you can't seem to get a handle on your nibbling, stop what you are doing and commit to doing ten minutes of yoga. Set a timer. When the bell rings, reassess your hunger level. It's likely that you'll feel a lot calmer and more in charge of the urge to eat. Keep in mind that you don't have to do these poses perfectly.

- **Cross-legged pose.** Try learning just one simple yoga pose. Become an expert on it. When you're in a bad mood or find yourself on the verge of an emotional eating binge, try the *sukhasana* pose, also known as the perfect pose. Essentially, this is sitting in a cross-legged position. Think about how easily this way of sitting came to you as a child. Once you get into this position as an adult, think about how it makes you feel. It's highly likely that you will need some time to relearn this position. You may notice yourself crossing your legs and working to find a comfortable position. Sit in this position for five minutes. Focus on your breathing. Notice the posture of your body. Pay attention to how your sensations change over time while you sit there.

- **The warrior pose.** It takes a lot of courage and strength to fend off food cravings. Call in your inner warrior. This pose strengthens the entire body while improving self-control. Spread your feet about two feet apart. Place your right leg about one foot behind you. Then raise your arms so that they are parallel to the floor. Slowly bend your left knee until your thigh is parallel with the floor. Raise your arms over your head. Then gently and slowly lower your arms, with your left arm pointing straight ahead and your right arm pointing behind you, until your arms are parallel to the floor. Concentrate on a spot in front of you. Take a few deep breaths, lower your arms to your sides, and bring your legs together. Reverse the position with your right arm and leg forward. If these instructions are too complicated for you to follow, just freeze into a position that you imagine a warrior would take. If you want to learn more advanced poses or you want to see pictures, visit www.yogajournal.com.

24. sweating at the life gym

I don't have a lot of time to exercise and I'm not very good at it. But I have to admit that once I get started, I feel so great. When my daughter turned two, I actually got more exercise than I ever did in my life before. I didn't get it in a gym. It was simply constantly running after her. —Kim

If you don't already work out to soothe yourself, it's likely that getting enough exercise is a real challenge for you. You probably love the feeling you get when you do work out or when you go for a brisk walk. But you can't seem to motivate yourself to do it regularly, despite the emotional rewards. Moving your body releases a flood of feel-good chemicals, such as endorphins and neurotransmitters, that elevate your mood.

If you have blamed a lack of time and energy as the major hurdle to regular exercise, the good news is that you don't have to go to the gym to get the benefits of these natural, soothing chemicals. There are many effortless ways you can move your body that take very little time, sweat, or money. You don't have to go out of your way to get exercise. It's likely that you do get some exercise just from your normal daily activities. If so, it's important to be mindful of this and to acknowledge it.

A study by Crum and Langer (2007) looked at maids who didn't work out in a gym but got exercise doing their cleaning jobs. The only intervention the researchers made was to emphasize that scrubbing and cleaning is exercise. They educated the maids on how many calories are burned while doing jobs like scrubbing and dusting. Researchers also told the participants the many other ways this type of exercise benefited their bodies. The outcome was surprising. Participants lost weight, their blood pressure dropped, and they were found to be significantly healthier on several measures. Simply acknowledging their movement as exercise (rather than changing their behavior) led to significant health benefits. So the next time you run after your child on the playground or walk up two flights of stairs, pay attention to it. Say to yourself, "This is great exercise!"

~self-soothing technique~
Going to the Life Gym

Make a list of the natural, effortless ways that you can get exercise. You may not have thought of these activities as exercise because they don't take place in a gym. But activities like carrying bags of groceries up flights of stairs, running after kids, vacuuming, and transferring from a subway to a bus are all forms of exercise. After making your list, find ways to increase the physical intensity just a bit. For example, carry only one grocery bag at a time up the stairs to make more trips. Make extra trips to the copy machine. Plan an extremely romantic night to lengthen the time of vigorous sex.

Increase Your Heart Rate in Less Than Five Minutes

- Do forty jumping jacks. You may want to commit to doing them during commercials.

- Do fifty hula hoop circular motions. If you don't have a hula hoop, imagine having one around your middle and rotate your hips around.

- Lie on the floor, hold your legs up, and move your legs in circles, as though you are riding a bike, until you tire and can't keep your legs up in the air any longer.

- Dance to one entire song. Keep moving from the start to the finish of the song.

- Have sex. Any kind of sexual activity that leads you to become aroused releases mood-elevating chemicals in the body.

Each day that you exercise, put a sticker on a wall calendar. Code the stickers for different healthy behaviors—a blue star could signify walking, and a yellow sticker biking. Notice whether the frequency of your emotional eating drops when you increase the amount of exercise you get. Aim for at least thirty minutes of activity a day.

25. sleep on it

I work the night shift at the emergency room. When I get home, I'm all wound up from dealing with an endless stream of accident and critical patients. By the time I kick off my shoes at home, I'm physically and emotionally tapped out. Instead of going to bed, I have a very bad habit of staying up late, which leads to snacking. I circle my kitchen like an airplane stuck in a holding pattern. Then I sit in front of the computer and munch on pretzels trying to get out of my postwork funk. When I simply go to bed and don't binge, I wake up the next day totally refreshed and feeling like a rational human being again. If not, I'm cleaning out everything in the fridge. —Rhonda

We often underplay the value and necessity of sleep. Sometimes we even take pride in ourselves for how little sleep we can get by with. Sleeping is not only soothing, it's essential. Without enough of it, you can feel edgy, and you're much more vulnerable to uncontrolled eating. Sleeping also helps you to clear your mind. After a good night's sleep, you may notice that you have a fresh perspective on matters. In part, this may be due to interrupting a negative stream of thoughts.

Neuroscientists believe that sleep may help people process their feelings and remember facts. For example, if you take a test, you will remember more if you study and then sleep than if you were to stay up studying all night. Think about how this applies to emotional eating. It's likely you will think more clearly and feel less emotionally wound up in the morning. A clearer head equals more balanced eating.

Getting a good night's sleep can even help you manage your waistline (Jones, Johnson, and Harvey-Berino 2008; Marshall, Glozier, and Grunstein 2008). The two hormones that control appetite are called leptin and ghrelin. When your sleep is too short, these hormones become unbalanced. Sleep-deprived people tend to have low amounts of leptin and high amounts of ghrelin. This leads to an increase in appetite. The imbalance, due to shortened sleep, may contribute to obesity. So getting a good night's sleep may not only help your mood, it may also help stabilize your appetite.

~self-soothing technique~
Mindfully Accept Sleep

- When you consider trying to get more sleep, do you say to yourself, "I have too much to do"? If so, work on giving yourself permission to sleep more. Sleep actually regenerates your body and will make you feel refreshed and more productive. Mindfully accept the need for sleep, even if it doesn't fit well into your plans.

- Consider that seven to nine hours of sleep a night is optimal (Jones, Johnson and Harvey-Berino 2008). Fewer hours than that, and you may be putting yourself at risk for stress eating and increasing your weight.

- If you have the urge to eat, try to take a quick catnap to recharge your batteries.

- Check in with your body. Are you low in energy? Do you want to eat to give yourself a little boost? Emotional eaters often turn to food for comfort when they are low in energy. Think about whether more sleep would give you the kind of energy you are seeking from food.

- If you don't have time to take a nap right now or you aren't close to a bed, just fold your arms and put your head down on your desk. Allow yourself to rest your mind for a moment. Breathe deeply.

- If you have trouble sleeping, try valerian tea, which is reputed to help people sleep. (But do check with your doctor to make sure it's okay.)

26. soak away stress

There is a well-known saying "When all else fails, take a bath."
This is pretty good advice. At night, taking a soothing bath
is now part of my routine instead of munching on peanuts and
Fritos. The bubbles and warm water melt away my stress much
better and for longer than snack foods. If I'm thinking about food
when I step in the shower, by the time I'm done, all such thoughts
are gone. —Jill

Hydrotherapy has been around since the time of the ancient Romans. They built bathhouses for bathing as well as for healing physical ailments. Heat and water are two of nature's most powerful healers. When they are blended together, they do a great job at gently massaging and relaxing the body.

Not only does a hot shower or tub feel great, it has clinical benefits. The medicinal power of hot tubs has been explored (Cox, Bernstein, and Hooper 2000), patients with type 2 diabetes used a hot tub thirty minutes a day, six days a week. After only ten days, they reported that they'd lost weight, needed smaller doses of insulin, slept better, and felt an increased sense of well-being.

In addition to the physical benefits, a bath or shower is often within easy reach and offers a private space to reenergize. Rarely do people dare to bother you there. However, many people don't get the full emotional benefits of a soothing shower because they bring their problems right into the shower stall with them, instead of checking them at the door. They may be among those who can cry only in the privacy of their own bathroom. They use the shower to hide their feelings rather than to wash them away.

If this sounds like you, consider taking a new kind of a bath, a mindful bath.

~self-soothing technique~
Taking a Mindful Bath

A mindful bath is one that you take alone, not with the hundred concerns you have.

- As you scrub, try to stop replaying ever worry and problematic conversation in your mind. Instead, allow yourself to be keenly aware of what is happening to your body. Focus on the drops of water on your arms. Inhale the aroma of the soap. If you see your mind being drawn back into your list of daily stresses, just bring your thoughts back to the moment by focusing on physical sensations.

- Before you step into the bath or shower, gather up some soothing bath lotions, bath salts, and oils. Bubbles, particularly scented ones, trap the scents. These bubbles send calming aromas to the brain. The olfactory nerve is closely connected to the limbic system, the part of the brain that manages emotion. This means that if you send pleasant scents to your brain, they are likely to stimulate soothing feelings.

- If it is hard to let go of your worries, it may be helpful to use imagery. As you massage the shampoo into your hair, imagine washing away your negative thoughts.

- We all unwind in different ways, especially when submerged in water. Create a soothing ritual. Play the same music. Get a fluffy, white robe to relax in after your bath or shower.

- Instead of a taking bath, create your own facial steamer. Put hot water into a bowl. Place your face over the bowl at a safe distance, then drape a towel over your head to trap the steam rising from the bowl of hot water. Leave yourself enough ventilation to breathe comfortably.

- If it's the middle of the day and taking a shower is simply impossible, head to the bathroom and place your hands under warm water for a minute. Focus your mind on the sensations of the water washing over your hands.

27. cleaning out the urge to eat

Most people think cleaning is a terrible chore. But scrubbing and organizing is incredibly soothing to me. I have an endless number of drawers to organize. It feels very productive and it takes my mind off the Twinkies that are hanging out in my cupboard. —Jenna

For the purposes of soothing, the point of cleaning is to keep yourself busy, give yourself a productive project that will give you a sense of accomplishment, and get your body moving. Notice this is not about having a spick-and-span house or having things clean and perfectly in order. The goal is to get your body and mind engaged in an active and rewarding project.

Housework can be exhausting when you have a long list of chores to do, you feel you must do it all, or it's intended to please other people. This cleaning technique is about helping yourself and no one else. It's not to get things done or even to get the house clean, but to help you cope with whatever is driving you toward food.

~self-soothing technique~
Scrub Away Stress Eating

- Make an emergency cleaning box. It's frustrating to have to look for a sponge when you are trying to stop emotional eating.

- Organize a closet or a drawer in your desk. Pick one small project. If you choose too large an area, you might feel overwhelmed and therefore could feel worse.

- Determine what kind of cleaning you enjoy. Maybe you hate to wash windows but love to iron because you can stand in place. Perhaps you like to sweep quietly but dislike vacuuming because it is too loud. If you are a detail person, scrubbing tile may be the way to go, instead of tossing a big load of laundry into the washer.

28. turn off the carnival in your head

When I'm overwhelmed with life, I am a champion stress eater. I get into this mood where I don't care what I am eating. I actually do care, later, but I don't have the emotional energy to make one more decision. Eating helps me to tone down my anxiety. Since I will never be free of daily hassles, I have to find a way to cope with it. Shutting off my cell phone, for example, for even an hour, helps me to slow down and gives me some time alone to recharge. —Carrie

Imagine you are driving a car. Suddenly, you realize you've made a wrong turn. What is one of the first things you might do, even unconsciously? It's likely you will turn off the radio. You try to reduce every kind of extra stimulation and distraction. Will this help you find the turn you should have made? It's not likely. But turning off the radio reduces the clutter your brain must sort through to focus on finding the right turnoff.

You might fall into the trap of stress eating because you feel overwhelmed by everything going on around you. If you cringe each time your cell phone rings or when you hear loud music, your body may be on overload. When your senses are constantly in use and are continually processing information, overstimulation results. Your eyes and ears don't have a chance to rest. Eating may be a way of trying to temporarily tone down or drown out the barrage of sensations you experience during the day.

Overstimulation is a common problem among young infants. People who play with babies often overdo it with cooing and singing too close to the child's face. A baby often averts his or her eyes from an adult's to gain a quiet moment. Teenagers are also vulnerable to being overstimulated. Too many flashy video games, lights, and gadgets with bells and whistles can make their brains a little dizzy. Both children and adults can benefit from giving their senses a rest. Doing that can help you to focus and to soothe yourself.

~self-soothing technique~
Switching to Shutdown Mode

When you feel overwhelmed, remove as much stimulation as is possible. This helps you to reduce the number of items your brain has to identify and sort through:

- The next time you realize that you are feeling overwhelmed, move to a quieter place.

- Be unreachable. Turn off your cell phone. Shut down your e-mail.

- Be mindful of your caffeine intake. Your system can be overstimulated by drinking too much caffeine. Caffeine can also cause you to feel wired or jittery.

- Imagine being a human statue. Be very still.

- Turn down all of your senses. Begin by turning off the lights. Cover your head with a pillow. Lower the shades. If you can't control the lighting, just close your eyes. Simply removing the visual cues to your brain eases its load a little.

- Unplug anything that makes noise. Turn off the radio. Find a quiet place. If it isn't silent enough, find a quieter place, even if it's only the stall of a bathroom. This is often a great place to recharge, as no one will bother you there.

- Remove any strong smells. If you can't get rid of strong odors, try taking a sniff of something pleasant, like a green apple, a cup of coffee, an orange peel, or a drop of vanilla.

- Change your clothes to something softer. Put on a cozy sweater. Your clothing might not be comfortable. Put on something loose and flowing.

- Put on a pair of headphones. Even if you don't have music on, people will leave you alone when you are wearing them.

- Go somewhere very quiet, like a library or a museum, or just sit in your car with the radio turned off.

- Use your hands to block external stimulation. For a minute, place your thumbs over your ears. With your thumbs still covering your ears, use your index fingers to cover your closed eyes. Sit that way for several minutes.

29. self-hypnosis

Unlocking the mystery of why I emotionally eat has been a challenge. There are so many reasons. The best thing for me is to not even ask why and just focus on stopping it in its tracks. Sometimes I do self-hypnosis. Basically, this is just a way of talking to my body and telling it how to relax. —Kayla

If you have ever done any relaxation training or yoga, you may also be a fan of self-hypnosis techniques, like progressive muscle relaxation. Basically, self-hypnosis is verbally walking yourself through detailed instructions on how to relax your muscles and your whole body.

Progressive muscle relaxation involves tightening and relaxing specific sets of muscles in a series. Try it briefly for a moment. Make a fist and squeeze tight. Hold the fist for at least ten seconds. When you let go, you will notice the change in tension. This technique works because you are forcing the muscle to become tense and then relaxed. When you force your muscles to become tense, they return to a more relaxed state than when you started. Then those muscles send signals to the rest of your body to also move into a more relaxed state.

~self-soothing technique~
Progressive Muscle Relaxation

Start with the top of your head and work your way down your body. Consciously place your attention on each part of your body as you tense and relax it. Feel the way your body seems to sink down as you release a muscle or a group of muscles.

1. Get comfortable. Sit with your feet flat on the floor, or you can lie on the floor. Breathe deeply.

2. Start at the top of your head. You will be tensing and relaxing the muscles around your face. Squeeze your eyes closed tight for a minute. Hold it. Then relax them.

3. Clench your jaw. Hold. Relax.

4. Tense your shoulders. Hold. Relax.

5. Feel your hands. Clench your fists. Hold. Relax.

6. Squeeze your buttocks. Hold. Relax.

7. Feel your upper legs and thighs. Tighten your muscles. Hold. Relax.

8. Feel your knees. Tense the muscles around them. Hold. Relax.

9. Clench your toes. Hold. Relax.

When you have progressively relaxed your body, mentally scan it to see if any part of you is still tense. If so, repeat tensing and relaxing that part.

~self-soothing technique~
Warming and Calming Your Body

Try a mini exercise similar to autogenic training, which is a technique for relaxing your body (Setter and Kupper 2002). When you give yourself these verbal commands, try to turn the words into pictures in your mind. Sit comfortably. Close your eye if you like. Breathe deeply. Focus on sensing what you are telling your body to feel. Say the following statements to yourself slowly, and try to feel the sensations you are instructing your bodily parts to feel.

My right arm is heavy.
My left arm is heavy.
My right leg is heavy.
My left leg is heavy.
My neck and shoulders are heavy.
I feel calm and peaceful.
My right arm is warm.
My left arm is warm.
My right leg is warm.
My left leg is warm.
My neck and shoulders are warm.
I feel calm and peaceful.
My forehead is warm.
My stomach is warm and full.
My stomach feels warm and satisfied.
My heartbeat is calm and regular.
I feel calm and peaceful.

Repeat the entire sequence as many times as you like.

30. be your own masseuse

Dao yin is a part of Chinese medicine. Basically, it's self-massage. When I do it, it helps me restore balance in the parts of my body that feel tight or achy. When I get into the self-massage techniques, I can feel the blood flowing and I feel calm—much calmer than when I stress eat. —Eric

If we could all make appointments at a spa for a therapeutic massage, that would provide most of us with an ideal soothing technique. Unfortunately, most of us can't do that as often as we would like. And you need the benefits of massage in the moments when you are wrestling with emotional eating, not at the time of your massage appointment. Luckily, you can do self-massage and get many of the same benefits. You may already do some form of self-massage and not understand that this is what you're doing. For example, if you have a headache, you might rub your forehead where it hurts. Or if you had a tough day, you might kick off your shoes and rub your feet.

For massage to be truly effective, you must be mindful of your body. Tune in to the spots that need comfort and healing. Do your shoulders feel tight? Is any part of your body in pain? Which part of your body needs soothing? The nice part of doing self-massage is that you are in control of the pressure applied. You can explore your body at your leisure and discover what truly feels good to you.

Massage therapy provides several important health benefits, such as improved blood circulation, reduced muscle tension, and relaxation. It also lightens your mood by providing you with stress relief and increasing your levels of endorphins or other biochemicals that make you feel good.

~self-soothing technique~
Be Your Own Masseuse

If physical discomfort is at the heart of your emotional eating, try some of these techniques. You may find that by addressing your physical discomfort, your desire to eat for emotional reasons has diminished.

- **Hands.** You will need some lotion for this technique. After you apply a dab of lotion to your hand, rub the palms of both hands together. Observe that some heat is created by the rubbing. Then clasp your hands together. Your fingers should be entwined. With your thumb, massage the area just below your other thumb in a circular motion. Continue massaging and move outward to the center of the palm. Rub each hand for two minutes.

- **Feet.** This exercise can be done standing or sitting. To massage your feet, you will need a hard beach ball, golf ball, or tennis ball. If you are standing, be sure to hold the edge of a chair for support. Place one foot on the ball. Then roll your foot back and forth over the top of the ball. Next place the arch of your foot on top of the ball. Apply pressure gradually. Roll the ball around under your arch. Then roll the sole of your foot. Finally, roll under your toes and your heel. Follow the same procedure for your other foot.

- **Shoulders.** You can also use a tennis ball for massaging your shoulders. Place the ball against a wall behind your shoulders. Roll the ball back and forth over and between your shoulder blades until you feel your shoulders relax. Do this for approximately three to five minutes.

- **Eyes.** Do you feel tension in your eyes? Briskly rub your palms together. As you rub, your palms will become warm. Then quickly, and gently but firmly, cover your eyes with your palms. Keep your eyes covered for half a minute. The warmth of your hands will transfer to your eyes.

- **Ears.** Using your thumbs and index fingers, begin by gently rubbing your outer ear rims. Then rub your earlobes. Continue doing this until your ears feel warmer.

- **Face.** For massaging your face, use the knuckles on your thumbs. Gently rub both thumbs' knuckles up and down alongside your nose, massaging up and down. If you want gentler pressure, do this with your fingertips. Then rub circles around your eyes with your fingertips. Make the circles large enough to completely reach around your eyes and above your eyebrows.

- **Head.** Rest both elbows on a table. Place your fingertips on your scalp underneath your hair. Massage your head with your thumbs and fingertips.

- **Stomach.** It's a natural response to rub your stomach when you overeat. Using clockwise, circular motions, rub your hand or palm over your abdomen approximately twenty times. Clockwise is the same direction that food travels in your intestines. This type of massage aids your digestive processes.

6 soothing yourself with distractions

In terms of stress or emotional eating, you can use mindfulness skills to help you cope by focusing on whatever is bothering you in an open and curious way. So some might think that distraction is the exact opposite of mindfulness. But in this context, distraction means something quite different. When you want to eat for emotional or stressful reasons, distracting yourself means to actively focus your attention on something other than food.

When you distract yourself, you are not avoiding or escaping your feelings as you do when you act mindlessly. *Distracting yourself* means to strategically divert your attention away from an emotional situation to a more neutral activity. It can be a very helpful coping skill when you can't seem to free yourself from stress eating.

Distraction is especially helpful if you are not truly physically hungry. Engaging your mind in another activity can help you be less caught up in negative emotions. Distraction can help you step aside and pause for a moment to observe how you are feeling. Sometimes distracting yourself can even physically take you away from the vicinity of food. If you are swimming, you can't dive into a box of crackers. Active behaviors remove the option of eating. You can also distract yourself with daydreams and simply choosing to think about something else that is soothing.

Distraction is especially helpful when it takes place *before* you engage in eating, rather than while you are consuming food. Note that distracting yourself while you eat a meal can actually increase the amount you consume (Bellisle and Dalix 2001). For this reason, reading and eating at the same time is not a wise idea. The kind of distraction techniques discussed in this chapter should be implemented as soon as you become mindful of the desire to emotionally eat.

31. emotional Band-Aids

Sometimes I don't know if I eat because I want the food or if it just feels good having something to chew on. The pencils on my desk are completely chewed down to stubs. Popping a fruity piece of gum into my mouth often helps curb my desire to munch on a donut. I'm glad I'm not a smoker or I would be smoking like a chimney. I am constantly putting something into my mouth. Now it's just a matter of chomping on things that don't make me gain weight. —Monica

For some emotional eaters, consuming food feels good for the pure act of eating. The bottom line is that putting something sweet or chewy in your mouth is enjoyable. The sensation of chewing is both stimulating and calming. If Freud were alive today, he'd have a thing or two to say about this. He'd call this need to self-soothe by eating an "oral fixation." According to Freud, the oral phase of development takes place during the first eighteen months of life.

If you've ever had a child, you know that everything goes into a baby's mouth at this stage. Infants explore the world through tasting and touch. Freud believed that if this developmental stage is not appropriately resolved (that is, if the child is weaned from the breast or bottle too early or too late), it sets up the child to become obsessed with putting things into his or her mouth later in life, whether it be cigarettes or food. Oral fixations are thought to contribute to problems related to the mouth, such as overeating, being overly talkative, having a smoking addiction, overindulging in sugar, chewing on straws, and having an alcohol addiction. Other symptoms include a sarcastic or biting personality, in which people become verbally hostile using their mouths. One might think that Freud's theory is a bit simplistic, as there are many psychological, social, and biological factors that contribute to all of these issues. Regardless of such criticism, we do know that sometimes the act of chewing can be pretty calming.

~self-soothing technique~
Soothing Chewing

- Try chewing on something that isn't food related, such as a breath mint, a stick of gum, a straw, or even your pen if nothing else is handy.

- One of the easiest ways to cope with a strong oral fixation is to drink plenty of liquids. Keep an eight-ounce, refillable water bottle beside you. Continue to refill it. The water (or other liquid) should help to calm your mood. Consider that your body is primarily made of water. When you add water, you're restoring the natural balance. Skip the coffee, tea, or caffeinated sodas. They deplete your body of water rather than adding to it. You can also try sucking on an ice cube.

- You may want to get a chew stick from the health food store. They come in many different flavors. They replace the eating behavior, and it's claimed that they're good for your teeth and gums. They may also help people quit smoking.

32. shop, drop, and roll

I've earned it. That is what my mind tells me about eating the cupcake sitting in front of me. I'm a good person. I work hard. I deserve this cupcake. This is a dangerous way of thinking that walks me right into emotional overeating all the time. —Mimi

In times of economic distress, economists refer what is called "the Lipstick Indicator." Historically, during a downturn in the economy, there is a noticeable rise in lipstick sales. Buying a lipstick is an easy, affordable way for women to get a quick pick-me-up that can brighten their day because it doesn't break the bank or cause weight gain.

If you eat food to reward yourself or to indulge or pamper yourself, you may want to consider shopping as an alternative. Some people have called buying things just to feel good "retail therapy." Buying something new can give you a little rush. Making a purchase actually raises levels of *dopamine*, which is the neurotransmitter in the brain that governs pleasure, satisfaction, and excitement. However, a word of caution here: Shopping can become a dangerous habit. It is still using something outside of yourself to provide comfort, rather than calming yourself with positive thoughts or actions. Also note that shopping can be just as addicting and damaging (to your wallet) as too much food can be to your appearance and health.

The positive aspect of retail therapy is that just getting out of the house and browsing can sometimes help distract you and take you away from the vicinity of food. Also, online shopping makes it possible to shop at any time of the day. If you're pacing the floor at night trying to avoid eating a midnight snack to take the edge off your mood, you can go shopping at your computer in your pajamas.

~self-soothing technique~
Find Your Lipstick Factor

Make a list of small, affordable pick-me-ups that have nothing to do with food. Your list could include a small bottle of lotion, your favorite gum, a new tool, a pair of sunglasses, a paperback book, or a song from iTunes. A new lipstick or lip balm (if you aren't a lipstick wearer) isn't a bad idea. It soothes your lips. When you feel the urge to eat, get out the lipstick (or lip balm) and apply some to your lips.

When you're about to engage in boredom eating or you need to distract yourself, try window shopping. Mindfully browse. You don't have to buy anything. Go to www.ebay.com or peruse books on www.amazon.com.

33. brain candy

I ride a train to work. I used to take a sack filled with food and eat it during my hour's commute. It kept me entertained. On the days I had to give a presentation and dreaded going to work, I nervously ate the entire time. Now I pack my iPod full of movies. I can stop and start the films at any time. Sometimes I can't wait to get onto the train to finish up the movie. It's a heck of a lot better than filling my time with eating salty snack foods and candy. —Katie

To the brain, movies are like candy because they stimulate the senses so intensely. They flood the brain with complex images, sounds, lighting, and dialogue. If your brain is stuck on food, being inundated with a movie's stimulants can help to dislodge the desire for food. Many clients refer to various movies during their counseling sessions. They talk about the characters that have inspired them, and sometimes they model the way various characters from films cope with difficult life situations.

Many of my clients have also shared the ways in which they connect with certain movies on a deeper level. For example, Katie revealed a connection with Jenny from *Forest Gump*. Jenny, an abuse victim, spent many years damaging her body and spirit with drugs and abusive relationships with men. Although Katie's issues weren't an exact copy of Jenny's, there were many things about Jenny's life that were familiar to Katie. She too had engaged in many years of self-sabotage.

When she watched *Forest Gump*, Katie sobbed uncontrollably. She had harmed herself with food and let her damaged self-esteem guide her choices. Seeing those choices unfold on screen helped her to recognize the forces that were driving her emotional eating and weight gain. A truly good work of filmmaking can make you laugh and cry. It can tap directly into your deepest emotions and reveal them to you.

~self-soothing technique~
Movie Therapy

- Watching movies often requires a chunk of time. If you are technically savvy, download a few movies onto your iPod or get a portable DVD player.

- Here are the names of some books that may help you find a movie to match your mood: *Cinematherapy for the Soul: The Girl's Guide to Finding Inspiration One Movie at a Time*; *Reel Therapy: How Movies Inspire You to Overcome Life's Problems*; and *E-motion Picture Magic: A Movie Lover's Guide to Healing and Transformation*. Most likely they are available from your local library.

- If you can't get any of these books, think about your favorite movie. What was the most recent film that lifted your spirits? What did you like about it? Ask a rental store to recommend a similar type of movie.

34. knit it out

Knitting is my new passion. I never tried it despite my grandmother's repeated attempts to teach me. My grandmother always had a ball of yarn in her lap. As a child, I was mesmerized by the movements of her hands. As a teenager, I thought knitting was very uncool and old-fashioned. I never dreamed that I would pick up the same habit as a way to soothe myself when I wanted to overeat. It's impossible to eat and knit at the same time. But it's more than that. When I'm knitting, I calm down right away. I wander into the kitchen to munch on food much less often than I used to do. —Regina

Expert knitters talk enthusiastically about the therapeutic and intoxicating nature of knitting. This craft can be so absorbing that many knitters can do it for hours on end. The sound of the clicking knitting needles and the movement of the hands does wonders to help clear the mind.

Dr. Herbert Benson, the founder and president of Harvard's Benson-Henry Institute for Mind Body Medicine and the author of *The Relaxation Response* wrote that knitting is soothing because it's a type of meditation (Benson 2001). In fact, the quiet, repetitive motions can induce the relaxation response. The relaxation response is the same set of reactions that occur when you meditate, are mindful, or do yoga. The body goes into a resting, relaxed mode that decreases heart rate and respiration. This may explain why some knitters rave about the soothing quality of knitting.

Not only is knitting physically soothing, but when you finish, you have something for your labor—a scarf, a baby hat, a blanket, or a sweater. If you knit a blanket, you may find yourself snuggling under it as it grows. Knitting is a soothing skill that you can take with you. Just stuff yarn into your carryall and pull it out anywhere you go.

~self-soothing technique~
No More Idle Hands

- Sign up for a knitting class. Look for knitting socials at local craft and yarn stores.

- If you don't have a class close by, you can seek instruction on the Internet or buy a book that demonstrates knitting techniques.

- If knitting is too difficult or you don't have time to learn, you can substitute any kind of stitching, such as cross-stitch, crocheting, embroidering, or simply braiding yarn.

- If knitting or crocheting is not for you, find another hobby with the same goal in mind—to keep your hands occupied and moving.

35. make a bucket list

Eat Thai food in Thailand.
Write a steamy romance novel.
Live in Colorado.
Learn Italian.
Make up with my ex-boyfriend.
—Ella

The sentences above are a few examples from my client Ella's bucket list. Ella named her list after the movie *The Bucket List*. It's about two men, both terminally ill, who go on a road trip together. They create a list of activities they want to do before they "kick the bucket." Since she made her list, whenever Ella has the urge to soothe herself with food, she reads it and thinks about her desires. Sometimes she adds another goal as a way to distract herself. It's fun and she easily gets caught up in daydreaming about her positive desires.

The idea of a list of things you want to do before you die may sound a little morbid. But creating this kind of list is a great distraction technique. It's an activity that requires only a pen, a piece of paper, a creative and active imagination, and some soul-searching. The main point of making such a list is to help yourself see the big picture. If you're struggling with emotional eating, you may be fixated on the present moment, on feeling good in this instant, or on immediate gratification. You may be attached to the idea that you really want to eat this food or you won't survive. But when you start to look at what you really want from life, these extra mouthfuls of food are not going to meet your needs, nor will they bring you satisfaction for the rest of your life.

A bucket list is a reminder of what is truly satisfying and what you really want from life. It's guaranteed that whatever you were planning to nibble on just a minute ago isn't going to make your top ten list.

~self-soothing technique~
Make a Bucket List

If you feel the urge to eat, pause for a just a moment. Ask yourself, "What do I really want from my life?" Then make your list. Or you might answer the following questions mentally. These topics will help to get you started on your list:

- I want to travel to…

- I want to accomplish…

- The hobbies I want to try…

- The thing I've never done that I'd like to try…

- What I would do only once would be…

- I wish my family could…

Next, pick something from your list and start planning how to make it happen, even if you aren't ready to do it immediately. For example, if you want to take piano lessons, look through the phone book for piano teachers. If you want to go scuba diving in Greece, look on the Internet for organized trips. Investigate where they go and how much they cost. This will not only distract you from thoughts about food, it will motivate you to start thinking about the steps you'll need to take to make your goals happen.

36. crafty ways to self-soothe

If I didn't have to work, I'd spend my day cooking, trying new recipes, and making batches of buttercream icing. I love to create new gourmet meals and to bake homemade bread. This passion doesn't help my waistline. If I was ever going to get a handle on my eating, I had to find something that tapped into my creative juices just as much as cooking does. —Joan

Joan was one of my best-dressed clients. Every week she'd come to therapy wearing an amazing outfit. I'd overhear the receptionist compliment Joan's "look." The secret to Joan's style wasn't expensive clothing. It was her homemade jewelry. Her necklace and earrings complimented the color of her shirt to perfection.

Joan didn't wear her jewelry for the compliments. She was the first to admit that making the pieces was her favorite form of personal therapy. Creating a work of art that she could wear each week made her feel good about her body. She focused less on her weight and more on her style. The process of stringing little beads on a nylon strand kept her hands too busy to pick at food. Also, planning the patterns took a lot of mental energy that pushed food to the back of her mind.

Creating things stimulates your brain in new ways. Designing patterns or seeing a work of art come together is both invigorating and challenging. Working at a craft can help you feel more excited and motivated in ways that simply relaxing may not. You may even observe that when you share your creations with others, you feel like a more well-rounded and interesting person.

Ironically, many emotional eaters are fantastic bakers. Because they love food, they may spend a lot of time baking and cooking. Although the action of cooking can be very soothing, it's also a recipe for a setup unless you focus on creating only healthy recipes! Very few cooks can prepare food without eating it. So instead of cooking to soothe yourself, try experimenting with some crafts.

~self-soothing technique~
Creative Soothing

- Create a craft nook in your home. Here are some of the crafts you can try out: jewelry making, painting, pottery, scrapbooking, candle and soap making, card making, sewing, and making homemade ornaments for holidays. You can use the time you would have spent on fixing and eating snacks for your creative time.

- Set up a routine time to do your creative pursuits. For example, you could designate every Saturday morning to mold clay or make soap. These creative endeavors can help you blow off steam and redirect your focus to something positive. You may start looking forward to Saturday mornings. Just thinking about the weekend approaching will be calming.

- Start a large, ongoing project. Have it be something that you can do a little at a time in your spare moments. For example, put together a family photo album. When you get the urge to snack mindlessly, try gathering and organizing photos instead.

37. exploring cyberspace

I was so bored I didn't know what to do with myself. The white chocolate macadamia cookies in the kitchen were beginning to call my name, loudly. If I didn't do something soon, I'd inhale them all, like a vacuum cleaner, in a matter of seconds. So I sat down in front of my computer and started looking up all the random things that crossed my mind. I don't have time to do this kind of investigation at work. This was the perfect moment to get lost in cyberspace. —Betsy

If you struggle with boredom, your computer offers you an endless possibility of distractions, from e-mail and instant messaging to iTunes and the Internet. Many businesses have chosen to ban Internet searches precisely because they lose a significant amount of productivity every day due to employees surfing the Web.

If you don't know where to start, try www.google.com and www.yahoo.com, which are two popular search engines. "Googling" has become known to many as a verb, as in one googles this or that topic. Searching the Internet will keep your mind and hands busy.

Type Away the Urge to Eat

- You could look up information about a person—someone you just met, the person you are dating, your neighbor, a high school classmate, your old college roommate, or your ex-boyfriend.

- Look up yourself. One of my clients calls this "ego-surfing." See whether there is any interesting information about you on the Web, or find someone who shares your name.

- Look up new equipment for your favorite hobby.

- Find travel sites.

- Look up the meaning of a word that you don't know.

- Try out www.youtube.com. Look for viral videos. *Viral videos* are the video clips that are so popular, they are sent around the world quickly—hence the name. Typically, they're pretty entertaining.

38. meditative music

Whenever I get into a bad mood, I skip right past the candy I have tucked away and head straight for my old Beatles' albums. In a matter of moments, I'm singing along, totally wrapped up in the music. Even if I was fighting some major cravings, they are gone as soon as I've played a song or two. There are certain songs I play when I'm down, like "Yesterday" and songs to pick me up, like "Love Me Do." A good song can make me feel better than a massage. —Judy

Certain songs can turn sadness to laughter, frustration to calmness, and anger to joy in only a matter of minutes. Lyrics contribute to the medicinal power of music. Think of a time when you heard a song that summed up perfectly how you were feeling. It's nice to know that someone has felt the same way that you have and has understood exactly how you feel. Music can also interrupt negative thoughts. Happy songs, for example, steer your mind in a more positive direction.

Music doesn't just calm your mind, it also impacts your body. Music has many therapeutic benefits because it affects the brain in so many complex ways. Certain types of music have been shown to enhance memory, calm mood, manage stress, alleviate pain, and improve communication. If you find a song soothing, you will know it by your breathing, which will slow down. Music therapists have also found that the movements of the heart muscles tend to synchronize to the beat of music. The rhythms of classical music are often similar to the average resting heartbeat of approximately 70 beats per minute. So listening to soothing music can help slow down a heart beating too rapidly, which may occur when you are anxious. Faster compositions stimulate your heart rate and sometimes they can actually speed up your entire nervous system.

~self-soothing technique~
Kick Back to a Soothing Melody

- Play some recorded music for at least twenty minutes. Or keep it on in the background to soothe you throughout the day. Don't know what kind of music to choose? Listening to your favorite music (or classical music) has been shown to reduce negative emotional states and physiological arousal much better than if you have no music playing or you are listening to heavy metal (Labbé et al. 2007). If you're a heavy metal fan, you may want to avoid it when feeling stressed. Aside from that, choose your favorite type of music to listen to when you are tempted to stress eat. It will provide you with a good distraction.

- If you are a musician, that's great too. If you are tempted to eat when you're not really hungry, play your instrument instead of reaching for food.

- Make a CD or an iPod playlist. Typically, premade CDs alternately mix fast and slow tempos. You may find it more helpful to keep the tempo the same, so that you don't feel calm during one song and ready to run a race when the next one comes on.

- If you want to be more mindful of how you feel, try listening to instrumental music without lyrics. Such music can help you be calmer and more contemplative. Song lyrics sometimes can get in the way of hearing your own thoughts.

- Energizing music is great for boredom eaters. Dance and get your body moving.

39. weeding out the urge to eat

Digging my hands into the dirt is so therapeutic. I work in an office, so I never get a chance to get dirty or to sit in the sunlight. Pulling out weeds feels so cathartic and rewarding. When I want to gobble up food, I go into the garden and start digging. It's harder to mindlessly chomp away at French fries when I'm reminded of how long it takes to hoe one row of potatoes.
—Diane

If you know someone with a green thumb, probably you've already heard about the therapeutic nature of gardening. Gardening has a number of soothing benefits that just might be what you are looking for.

Gardens bring forth your nurturing qualities. Flowers and vegetables require frequent care and tending. Maintaining a garden directs a person's awareness toward the notion of adequate care. Too much or not enough water can be harmful, just like eating too much or too little food. You must get to know your garden well to water it exactly the right amount. You also have to pay attention to the environment. After too much rain, you respond by reducing the amount of watering you do. Think about how similar this is to learning your own needs and to feeding your hunger appropriately. You too must continually adjust how much you eat.

If you keep plants inside your home or at your office, you are increasing the amount of oxygen in the air around you. The plants take in carbon dioxide and use it (with sunlight) to sustain life. Then they expel oxygen back into the atmosphere.

Mending and Tending Your Mood

- Gardening is an ongoing process. If it isn't the right time of year now, do some homework and plan your garden. Investigate seeds. Check out the varieties of vegetables in the grocery store and determine what you want to grow.

- Once you've got a garden, when you get the urge to eat, head outdoors and weed the garden. This work can be very soothing, particularly when you are stressed or angry.

- If you don't have room for a garden, try keeping a plant on your desk. When you feel the urge to eat, get up and water your plant first (if it needs it). Try taking care of its needs before your own. By the time you get back to your desk, observe whether your urge to eat has changed a little.

- Try growing an herb garden small enough to sit on your windowsill.

- Think about gardening in a symbolic way. Imagine pulling your negative thoughts out like weeds.

40. mini mental challenges

I love the taste of potato chips. I could munch away on them all day long. Mindless eating pushes me into this weird mental twilight zone. I don't really taste the chips. Nor do I think about how many I ate. When I'm sufficiently relaxed, I wake up from being zoned out and freak out about how much I ate. I try to just lie down instead of eating, but I get bored and feel lazy when I'm not doing anything. Recently, I've found other calorie-free ways to unplug. I've become addicted to puzzles! —Ariel

Ariel was about to take a test to become a certified dental assistant. If she didn't pass it, she wouldn't be hired by the local dentist who had promised her a job. She was feeling terribly worried. After hours of studying, she couldn't concentrate any longer. She couldn't stop thinking about what would happen if she didn't pass. Many disastrous scenarios raced through her head. She was very tempted to reach for the box of crackers on the desk. She could make them disappear in a heartbeat if she let herself.

Instead, Ariel took a mini mental break. She flipped through a puzzle book she'd bought at the magazine stand down the street. Ariel had picked it up only because her sister was obsessed with puzzles. She'd wondered what the attraction was. She chose a puzzle for beginners and got started. In a few minutes, she was completely immersed in the puzzle. She completely forgot her anxiety. The upcoming test vanished from her mind. When she'd finished the puzzle, she felt an huge sense of accomplishment. This gave her the needed boost to start studying again with a fresh mind. Puzzles are like exercise for the brain. They help develop new connections and use parts of the brain that are not always operating. Wouldn't it be nice to access more parts of your brain so that they can logically talk you out of stress eating?

~self-soothing technique~
Calming Mind Games

- Try puzzles like Sudoku and crosswords. You can print them from the Internet for free. Make sure to pick one at your level. If it is too easy, you will get bored quickly. Puzzles or games that are too difficult can cause great frustration, which doesn't help. Try to choose those exactly at your skill level.

- Print a few puzzles and keep them handy in the kitchen or in your desk. Place them anywhere tempting foods are kept or at your favorite places for mindless eating.

- Try easy computer games like solitaire, which is a card game you can play alone. Or get a jigsaw puzzle. It can keep you busy for hours.

- If you don't like games, try finding something else that might challenge your mind a little. Read an article from a magazine or listen to National Public Radio (www.npr.org).

Magnet Notes

It's likely that you have plenty of magnets on your refrigerator. We mostly use these helpful little gadgets in very functional ways—to hang little reminder notes and photos. Often, these magnets are the only things standing between you and opening the refrigerator. So why not use them to your full advantage? Buy a set of letter or word magnets. You'll find large collections on wordmagnets.com and thinkgeek.com. When you are tempted to open the refrigerator, spend a few minutes making up a sentence or poem. You'll be surprised at how addicting this action can be.

7 soothing yourself with social relationships

Connecting with friends and family is much more rewarding and healing than the comfort you can obtain from eating (Freeman and Gil 2004). The trick is to get the right kind of healing connection and support when you need it. Kind, supportive words from a soothing friend can make the difference between a food binge and calming down without having eaten one bite because of stress.

In this chapter, you will find healthy ways to reach out to comforting people for support. Don't be afraid to lean on these relationships during stressful times. If you don't have a great many friends or you are introverted, that's okay. It is not the number of people that heals but the quality and depth of your relationships. You can find these supportive connections in many different ways.

It's important to connect with the right people and to avoid toxic people. These are the friends and family members who try to guilt-trip you into doing things you don't want to do. They make you feel bad by being overly critical or by telling you you're not good enough. You may not be able to cut these people out of your life, but you can control how much time you spend with them and how much toxicity you allow into your life.

You need to find a good balance between self-soothing and being soothed by others. Friends and family members can provide you with helpful insights, cheerleading, and supportive statements. But you need to know how to calm yourself when you are alone. Also, you don't want to stress out friends by leaning on them too often. This chapter will also help you learn how to apply the soothing you've obtained from loved ones in your past to the present day. In other words, don't worry if you are alone or live far away from people who care about you. You can use some of these skills even when you are all alone.

41. the buddy system

I could go for two weeks without going for a run. But if I make a date to meet Victoria to go jogging, I will definitely be there. No excuses. No backing out. We help each other out all the time, and I don't want to let her down. I call her cell phone whenever I think I'm about to binge. I don't even have to say much. Just hearing her voice is enough to make me feel better because I know that she gets how I'm feeling. —Marie

Marie is someone who greatly benefits from the buddy system. She teamed up with her friend and coworker Chelsea. They make a great team. The two women support each other by venting their worries to each other. Despite very different lives, both women struggle with overeating and exercise. Marie is married and has a new baby. Chelsea is single and taking care of her ailing mother. They found a common bond in their challenges as primary caregivers. Daily, they discuss how difficult it has been to balance their own needs with those of their loved ones. Marie sends Chelsea supportive e-mails. Chelsea makes healthy slow-cooked meals that she shares with Marie's family. They often walk and talk, which helps to cut down on their emotional eating.

Ideally, like Marie and Chelsea, your buddy will be a friend who wants to help you and is also in need of emotional support from you. Often it's much easier for others to be empathetic when they understand your struggles personally or have lived with similar challenges.

Sometimes it is helpful to have more than one supportive relationship. If one buddy isn't available or is too busy with his or her own issues, it's beneficial to have another buddy to turn to. Moreover, one friend may be particularly good at cheerleading when you need encouragement, while another friend may be great at confronting you in a kind way when you slip up. Various relationships also bring forth different qualities and strengths from you.

~self-soothing technique~
Your Soothing Sponsor

- Choose your buddy wisely. Your buddy should be nonjudgmental and a good listener and shouldn't want to compete with you.

- Think of the person you choose as your soothing sponsor—someone who provides only support, not therapy or advice. Agree to call each other before engaging in emotional eating. As soon as you get the urge to emotionally eat, pick up the phone. Or if you are feeling vulnerable, call before you feel the urge.

- Chose a code word (a neutral word or phrase) to discreetly signal on the phone that you are in need of help.

- You also may want to come up with a motto or a slogan that exemplifies your goals. This can be a motivational quote or a team motto.

- Send your buddy encouraging words randomly by e-mail. Leave a thoughtful voice message. Send a poem by snail mail.

- Be a mindful listener. When you are with this person, let go of everything else on your mind. Try to avoid listening with just one ear or becoming distracted by your own thoughts. Really focus on everything your buddy is saying.

- Buy a copy of this book for your buddy and look through it together. Discuss which techniques might work well for the two of you to do together.

- Make each other accountable. Agree on the number of times you will check in with each other. Be proactive. Call instead of waiting for your buddy to call you.

- Meet regularly. For example, go for a walk every Tuesday night, call each other on Sunday evenings, or send a supportive e-mail every other day.

- Set good limits. It's okay to say no to each other when you need to.

- Give positive feedback as often as possible. When you want to do this, always start with a positive comment and follow it up with the issue you want to address. Be sure to give each other an equal amount of time to talk.

- Reward and celebrate positive changes together.

- If you can't find a buddy, try a pen pal or join an online virtual support group with people who are dealing with similar issues. Food problems are often influenced by one's culture, ethnicity, and environment. Writing or e-mailing to someone you don't know but who is from another background gives you something interesting to do. It also provides you with a sense of connection to a world larger than your own. And it helps you be mindful of how your culture and friends shape your issues with food.

~self-soothing technique~
Picture Someone You Love

Create a photo collage of comforting pictures for your desk or bedroom mirror—your child's first birthday, photos from your prom, a snapshot from a favorite vacation spot, and so on. Select photos that make you smile effortlessly. When you are struggling with food cravings, look at your collage or find a box of old photos to look through. Then put up these photos in places where you will be sure to see them when you get the urge to binge.

42. join the blogosphere

Every afternoon I check out the updates from my favorite bloggers. It's fun to read about the craziness, adventures, and ordinariness of someone else's life. Sometimes it makes my worries seem like small potatoes. Other times it helps me feel a little more normal. Sure, checking out someone's blog is a little voyeuristic, but it is very entertaining. It keeps me very amused during the moments I could be snacking. —Dawn

Blog is shorthand for Web log. These are Internet journals that are open to anyone to read. There is a blog for just about everything. There are even blogs about people who blog. Blogs give you a brief peek into someone else's mind. Before the Internet, people weren't privy to the private lives of people they didn't know and would never meet in person. Blogs have changed that. They're a great way to entertain yourself and ward off boredom eating. You can spend a lot of time online investigating how other people handle stress eating. Look for tips and advice. Reading about someone else's struggles with food really can help you understand your own. Such reading may give you a new perspective and remind you that you are not alone.

~self-soothing technique~
Blog It Out

Create your own blog. Use it as a way to process your feelings. The advantage of using a blog rather than a journal is that it's right on your computer desktop and can be easily tailored to meet your needs. If you don't feel comfortable sharing your feelings and viewpoints with the entire world, keep a private blog. Go to www.blogger.com to start a free site of your own. Give your blog a central theme, like "New Mom Struggling with Food Addiction" or whatever is bothering you.

If you aren't in the mood to share your thoughts, check out one of the many blogs already in cyberspace. There is sure to be a blog similar to your concerns or to what you would like to write about. Go to www.bloglines.com and www.technorati .com. Or enter "emotional eating" on the sites www.blogcatalog .com and www.mybloglog.com. A list of all the blogs already created about this topic will pop up.

A few words of caution: Be careful not to reveal too much personal information, such as your full or real name or where you live. Also, don't say hurtful things about other people. You can put yourself in danger. It is also considered unprofessional to reveal too much to others if you work with the public as a teacher or a counselor. Avoid giving too many identifying details. Also, be careful which sites you choose. There is a lot of harmful and inaccurate advice on the Web. You may want to start with blogs associated with universities, treatment centers, and health writers for newspapers or science journals.

Virtually Connect

Websites such as www.facebook.com, www.myspace.com, twitter .com, and www.myyearbook.com are some of the largest networking sites that allow you to connect with people in cyberspace. If you're already on one or more of these sites, it's likely that you've reconnected with old friends and even family members you haven't seen in a long time. You even may have found some new virtual friends. When you get the urge to emotionally eat, commit to sending at least one message (it doesn't have to be about food). Or look for one new friend. When you're done sending a message or have found a new buddy, reevaluate your hunger level.

43. helpful ways to vent

I tend to eat when I'm angry. If I can just vent my frustrations to someone, typically I feel better. Sometimes I use my journal to vent to myself. Other times I call my best friend. Letting off some steam is much healthier and more productive than stuffing my face with junk food. —Tina

Tina, a veterinarian, called her sister from her cell phone as she drove home from work. She told her sister all about the frustrating events of her day. She had been inundated with pet emergencies and one unexpected crisis after another. By the time she arrived home, she had run out of things to say and she felt much better. Just getting it off her chest was all she needed to calm down without the assistance of a sweet snack.

There are many different ways to vent. Some ways are helpful, some are not. Aggressive or traditional ways of venting, like throwing things or hitting a pillow, can sometimes increase rather than decrease your frustration and anger (Bushman 2002).

The type of venting that is helpful, and recommended, is putting how you feel into words. Basically, this means articulating your experience and emotions to another person. In part, it feels good to have someone listen. It makes us feel important and as though we have something worthy to say. Talking to someone also forces you to create a coherent story about your feelings. You take jumbled-up emotions and organize them in a way that make sense to someone else. When you vent, you explain to someone the reason something made you upset, which can lead to a lot of insights and aha moments.

A friend, coworker, or relative who allows you to vent is giving you a gift of their time and attention. They allow you to express yourself in a controlled and safe manner. Try to be mindful of this and open to their suggestions and perspective.

Take note that venting is different than problem solving. Basically, when you vent, you are not trying to fix the situation. Looked at realistically, some situations can be neither fixed nor changed. For example, you can't get rid of your boss, and neither can you change her. You must find a way to get along with her. Venting about her annoying habits may be your best option.

If you want venting to be helpful instead of hurtful, keep in mind that you need to be careful about whom you choose to vent to. The best person to unload your feelings to is a close friend or a trusted family member. Additionally, there are some important rules about whom you should never vent to. Many people have made the mistake of airing their grievances at work, only to be overheard by someone in management. Or your problems could be turned into office gossip. This just makes things worse. Another rule is not to vent to the person causing you grief. It's too easy for venting to feel like an attack, even if it isn't meant that way. This would defeat your purpose.

~self-soothing technique~
Venting Instructions

When you call a friend to vent, let him or her know immediately what you are asking for. Be specific. Start the conversation with "I'm so mad at myself for emotionally overeating. I'm calling because I need someone to…" This is where you fill in the blank. You may want a sympathetic ear, a cheerleader, or a reality check. Sometimes close friends think they have to fix your feelings or give you suggestions. However, the person listening to you vent need only listen, not give advice or try to change your situation.

If you don't have anyone to vent to, consider writing a letter to someone you might want to tell your grievance to. But don't mail this letter. Writing a letter is safer than sending an e-mail, especially if you don't mail it. It's too easy and too tempting to send e-mails. If this sounds too taxing, you can talk to a mirror. If you don't know how to begin, start by asking yourself this question: "What about this situation makes me so upset? Why do I feel that I need to get it off my chest?"

44. when you are all alone with a quart of ice cream

If I could call Marie, my best friend, at this moment, she'd tell me some harmless gossip, make me giggle, and keep me so amused that I'd forget about my stupid chocolate craving. But she has a big exam tomorrow and I don't want to bother her. Besides I need to do this myself. If she could just be attached to my hip at all times, I'd be fine. I hate that I use food as my stand-in for my best friend. —Amy

Sometimes it feels like there is no one and nothing to turn to except the ice cream in your freezer. It's 2:00 a.m. and your best friend is away on her honeymoon. Or perhaps you are new in town and haven't made any close friendships yet. There just isn't anyone convenient to turn to for support when you really need it. Food cravings don't wait for convenient moments. So what can you do?

This is when you have to get a little creative. Visualize someone who has done a good job of comforting you. It might be a parent, a friend, or a teacher. (Many teachers are skilled at reaching out to students with personal problems.) This person can be from your past or your present, and need not even be alive. Perhaps your grandmother was the most supportive person in your life. Although she has been gone for several years, you still miss her comforting skills and her ability to make you feel better. Or the person who provides the most comfort to you may be your therapist. If you are in therapy, perhaps you can guess what compassionate and empathetic words your therapist would use if you were sitting in his or her office talking about how uncomfortable you are feeling.

The necessary supportive words might come from someone you haven't really met, like a character in a book or a play. You may know the author's philosophy and values. For example, if you're a Jane Austen fan, you may have read enough of her work to be able to imagine how she would counsel you about the problems in your love life.

Most people internalize the voices of those closest to them. Often they're unconscious of the influence these voices have on the ways they comfort themselves. When I ask a client to imagine what a friend would say to cheer her up, often she can guess. For example, Linda said, "Yes, I know what my friend Sarah would say if I was depressed like today. She'd say, 'Girl, that's enough moping. Be ready in ten minutes. We're going shopping.'" My point is this: you don't need someone to be physically present to converse with him or her or to get the benefits of your friend's soothing.

~self-soothing technique~
Talk It Out

If you are having a hard day and no one is available to help you feel better without resorting to food, you can do this exercise in one of the following two ways:

- **Write it out.** Write a letter in a blue pen. Describe in vivid detail how you feel. Then take a different color to write a response. The response should be written from the perspective of a comforting friend or parent. The different color pen reminds you to stay in the other person's voice.

- **Role-play.** If you are a visual person, set an empty chair across from you. Imagine your friend sitting in that chair. You may even want to get up and sit in the chair, as if you were your friend. You may feel silly, but it's likely that you will get into the role of your friend after a few minutes. And if role-playing gets you to smile, would that be so terrible?

45. your furry friend and unconditional love

My dog is my best friend and my therapist. When he hears me open up the refrigerator, Lucky comes running. He gives me this look of deep concern. Lucky always knows when I'm having a hard time. I thank Lucky for watching out for me, and I stroke his coat until my futile food craving passes. His soft fur is soothing. I vent all my frustrations about food and how much I wish this problem would just go away. Lucky never rolls his eyes or stops listening like some of the people in my life. He also snuggles up close and never shies away from my touch. I don't know what I'd do without him. —Jackie

If you are having a hard day, there is no better medicine than snuggling up with man's best friend. This isn't just a good suggestion, it is scientific fact. Pets have great healing powers and incredible therapeutic value (Lilienfeld and Arkowitz 2008). This is great news given that half the homes in America have pets.

In addition to being your favorite buddy, a pet can be one of your best assets in finding comfort without resorting to food. If you are drawn to food because of a sense of emptiness, loneliness, or boredom, your relationship to your pet may be key to moving past this. You can have a very straightforward and uncomplicated relationship with a pet. No games. No name-calling. It is a reliable and safe friendship.

Noah, a recently divorced schoolteacher, realized that pets are excellent at listening and keeping secrets. When feeling angry with his ex-wife (who'd recently had an affair that had led to their divorce), he always talked it out with his dog. Rocky, Noah's dog, had an uncanny way of knowing how Noah felt. Rocky could sense Noah's despair and often tried to get Noah in a better mood. Like Noah, try to open up to your pet. It will help.

People who live with pets often talk about the social benefits that come with having a pet. For example, they often help you start conversations with random strangers. If you are having a food craving, hang out with your dog at the park and respond to people who talk to your pet. One of my clients brings her cat to family functions. The cat provides a great buffer and a diversion from family tensions.

~self-soothing technique~
Calming Moments with Your Pet

- When you are craving comfort foods, consider taking your dog for at least a ten-minute walk, if not longer. The exercise itself will help you to feel better. And spending some time with your dog or cat may give you the unconditional love you might really be craving.

- If you have a cat, keep a toy handy like a fishing pole, feather, or squeaking ball. There's nothing better to get your mind off your troubles than watching your furry friend happily bounce around with a toy.

- What if you don't have the energy to play to play with your pet? That's okay too. Simply holding or stroking an animal's coat can decrease your heart rate and lower your blood pressure. Find a cozy corner and commit to ten minutes of petting and talking to your pet.

- Pet owners know that pets, much like kids, require structure and routine. They need to be fed and walked about the same time every day. Use this to your advantage. If you are troubled by midafternoon snacking, keep yourself busy by taking your dog out for a walk or brushing your cat. Eat together at set times.

- If you don't own a pet, consider borrowing one. Offer to take your neighbor's dog for a walk or do an Internet search and start looking for a dog that needs to be walked.

- If you don't have a pet, you might consider getting one, but be sure to pick a pet that matches your personality and lifestyle. If you pick a pet that doesn't match you, it will be more stressful than helpful in your efforts to control mindless eating. Or go to an animal shelter to volunteer.

46. stepping into someone else's shoes

I saw a clip on TV of a woman who had bought a pair of Oprah Winfrey's shoes at a sale of Oprah's clothes. Whenever the woman felt blue or lonely, she put on the shoes and imagined what Oprah would do or say. It always worked to lighten her mood. I can see why this is helpful. I've taken acting classes that taught me the value of trying to look at the world through someone else's eyes. When I play someone very different from myself, like a motorcycle mama or a socialite, I study these characters closely. I try to understand who they are, what they think, how they feel, and their motivations. The techniques I learned in acting class help me cope with stress eating. I practiced being someone who doesn't struggle with food. I tried to understand and copy how such a person would behave. After a while, I wasn't acting, it was really me. —Melissa

Each day you observe people all around you to learn how to do certain things. Let's say that you go to a new restaurant. You may watch other people to determine if you are expected to seat yourself or wait for a hostess to escort you to your table. Or maybe you decide to stay at work past five o'clock because you see your coworker still sitting at her desk when it's time to go home. You can pick up a lot of helpful coping habits from observing others. Maybe you observe that your sister-in-law goes for a jog whenever she has a stressful day. Or your husband says humorously, "Oh well," whenever he makes an error. You can try on other peoples' coping skills for size.

~self-soothing technique~
Act It Out

Observe your friends, family, and coworkers for at least a week. Focus on positive role models who soothe themselves without food. Do research and ask them how they handle particular situations. Take a lot of notes. Write down what they say to themselves. Watch their body language.

Once you observe some coping behaviors, then you can try them out by using acting skills. Even if you don't have any particular acting talent, give it a try. Just mimic the healthy, effective ways you see that people use to calm themselves.

Here's another way you can use acting: When you're in a good mood, act out the ways in which you could avoid emotional eating successfully. For example, role-play walking into the kitchen and opening up the refrigerator as if you were about to stress eat, but then walk right out of the kitchen and engage in a distraction. The value of role-playing is in rehearsing the behavior so that it can become automatic. My clients often repeat the saying "Fake it 'till you make it." Sometimes you must do the behavior for a while before it becomes natural, familiar, and easy to do.

Mirror Image

Here's another way you can put your acting skills to good use. Put an empty chair across from where you're sitting. The two chairs represent your two conflicted sides: the side that wants to eat for comfort and the side that wants to eat only at scheduled mealtimes when hungry. Perhaps, at this very moment, you're feeling torn and conflicted about whether to dive into stress eating. Sit in one chair to make the argument for emotional eating. Then get up and sit in the other chair to argue against emotional eating. It's essential to get up and physically move from chair to chair. When you move your body and shift it to another location, it literally helps you to see things from another perspective. Notice how your mood changes as you shift into each role.

47. blockers for boredom eating

I love trying something new. This wasn't always so for me. I used to be phobic about change. I clung to the same old things, afraid I wouldn't like something new. Now I regret not being more open to things in the past. My narrow-mindedness made me miss a lot of opportunities. When a new idea pops into my mind, I no longer dig my heels in. This attitude has helped me to find creative ways to stop stress eating. —Jim

Do you eat out of boredom? If you try to nibble away the monotony of a dull half hour, it's important to try stimulating your brain in a different way. When you do something new, you actually change your brain chemistry. Sensations and experiences you've never encountered before create new neural pathways. Stimulating your brain in novel ways makes you smarter and helps you to think of more creative solutions to problems, including the issue of overeating. Doing something new is also challenging. It requires all of your focus. It's hard to stay bored when you try to acquire a new skill.

Trying out a hobby that you've never attempted before can also help you form new relationships. You may widen your social network by joining a new club or class. You may meet a teacher who can show you how to practice the new skill. You may make new friends. Trying something new, outside of your normal routine, provides you with entertaining stories to tell others, which can be useful when you want to socialize in order not to eat.

~self-soothing technique~
Try Something Novel and Innovative

There are few things worse than feeling that you are stuck in a rut. Doing something out of the ordinary can rev up your energy level. Before you get started, make sure you are in the right frame of mind. Don't be surprised if your mind plays tug-of-war between wanting to do something new and wanting to go back to the familiar. It is a natural human reaction to resist change. At first, remind yourself to keep an open mind, even if you don't like the new activity. Tell yourself, "Give it a try" and "Stick with it."

Not sure what new frontier to conquer? Here are some suggestions for new activities:

- Turn a new direction—literally. On your way home, make a left turn instead of a right. Take the scenic route around the neighborhood. Have you often wondered what was across the next avenue? Take a peek. Drive or take a walk on some unfamiliar roads.

- Find a new station on your radio to listen to. If you're a rock fan, try listening to the blues or to Spanish music. At first, you may not like it. Try to be open to the new sound. Don't change the station back to your tried-and-true programs immediately. Allow at least several songs to play.

- On your next trip to the grocery store, buy a vegetable or bread you've never tried before. Or purchase a familiar food but with a flavor you haven't sampled yet. For example, if you like salsa but always buy the mild, try something hotter.

- Shop for a new outfit. If you wear black all the time, try red. Try on something that doesn't "look like you" at all, such as a different style of shirt or cut of pants. If you're a jeans person, get a dressy outfit or a sexy pair of shoes.

- Investigate clubs in your community. Look for a biking club, a book club, an herb or gardening society, or a volunteer organization.

- Make something healthy from scratch—an applesauce cake, wine, or homemade granola. Find a recipe and go to town.

Remember that your overall goal is to stretch your comfort zone. You may need to think carefully about what is truly new for you and what is sticking to the old tried and true you know and love.

48. healing touch

What do I really need right now instead of a chocolate milkshake? A hug. I need someone to wrap her or his arms around me and tell me that it will be okay. When I get the desire to consume food like a human garbage disposal, I stop and ask myself what will really make me feel better. Nine times out of ten, I seek out my husband to wrap me up in a bear hug or rub my back. —Nelly

The next time you engage in comfort eating, think about the following study. It offers compelling evidence that snuggling will give you much more soothing than a chocolate brownie. Often, the touch of a hand and the warmth of an embrace will be the kind of comfort you are really seeking.

A very well-known study conducted in 1953 by psychologist Harry Harlow examined the importance of the sense of touch among animals. In the study, Harlow took baby rhesus monkeys away from their mothers. He then put them in a cage with two possible surrogate mothers. One mother was made of terrycloth, the other of wire. But the wire mother was able to provide food to nurse the babies. Time and again, when the baby monkeys were frightened, they ran to the terrycloth mother for comfort. Food wasn't nearly as soothing as the cuddly terrycloth mothers, even when the monkeys were hungry (Suomi, van der Horst, and van der Veer 2008).

Of course, there are differences between monkeys and humans. But this research demonstrated that the comfort all animals get from touch is a basic biological need. The Harlow experiments also indicated that the need for a comforting relationship and touch is as important as even the need for food.

~self-soothing techniques~
Warm and Fuzzies

- Give and ask for bear hugs. First, be sure to ask if it's okay. Hugging someone without permission may be a violation of his or her personal space and boundaries. A refusal of your touch or to hug back may feel very rejecting and ignite a further need for soothing within you.

- If you need a very gentle touch, ask for your back to be patted or the top of your hand rubbed.

- If you don't have anyone handy to cuddle with, try sandwiching yourself between two pillows. Or sink into a beanbag chair.

49. volunteer yourself

Once a month, I go to a local shelter and serve soup. My church asked for volunteers. Initially, I didn't want to do it. But after the first time I went, it changed my life. It put a thing or two into perspective for me. Instead of beating myself up for overeating food, I started being grateful that I had more than enough to eat. It encouraged me to consume food with a sense of appreciation instead of guilt. Also, I can't even describe how fantastic I feel when I leave. I feel like I have done something very important for people who truly appreciate it. I hardly ever feel that sense of gratitude from others or see people who are as happy to see me as those in the shelter are happy to see me. —Brad

Hollywood stars gain a lot of attention for their philanthropic endeavors across the globe. Big stars and minor starlets are photographed feeding hungry people in Africa and trying to forge diplomatic peace in countries where women and children's lives are in daily danger. What is this about? Is it just an effort to gain attention? In some cases that may be true. But I would venture to say that the reason is much deeper than that. Anyone who has volunteered to help those less fortunate knows that making a difference in another person's life is more gratifying than anything else one could possibly do. Money can only go so far to make you happy. It can entertain you for a while, but helping others changes your soul.

There's a philosophical debate about whether altruistic gestures—acts of helping others without asking for anything in return—are truly selfless acts. Why? Well, helping people gives you such a sense of personal reward that it's hard to make the argument that you get nothing back.

~self-soothing technique~
Give a Hand

If you are in an emotional funk and need to lift your spirits without resorting to food, find a way to give something of yourself.

- **Start small.** Give someone's self-esteem a little boost by handing out a compliment. Keep in mind that it must be genuine praise. Tell the cashier at the grocery store she did a great job of bagging your groceries. Compliment a coworker who looks especially nice. When you see the other person's face light up, you'll feel great.

- **Look to the people near you.** Volunteering is something we can do every day. It doesn't require going out of your way or very much time. Ask yourself what would help out—even a little. For example, you can offer to babysit for an hour. Or you can call your neighbors, and if they need something at the grocery store, offer to pick it up for them. Hold open a door for a woman carrying a baby or a man with his hands full. Carry an older person's groceries to his car. Buy a cup of coffee for someone who looks like she needs a break.

- **Look in the yellow pages.** There are many reputable service organizations you could work with in the phone book. Or you could try the Internet. Call local charities or social service organizations. You can also volunteer through your church or community center.

50. connecting even when you want to crawl under the covers

I just want to lock myself in my house and never come out. It is way too much effort to explain how I feel right now to anyone. The problem with barricading myself in my house is that I eventually get lonely and start going a little stir-crazy. Then I turn to food to entertain myself. I really am a social person and would probably feel better if I talked to someone. I just have trouble getting started. —Taylor

Although connecting with other people is extraordinarily healing, sometimes relating to others can feel like too much effort. In spite of the fact that you know talking to others will help, you may have no desire or motivation to connect. So, what do you do?

If being around people would help you to lessen your urge to stress eat but you just don't feel up to it, you can find ways to ease into interacting with others. Here are some helpful strategies to give yourself a little nudge out the door.

~self-soothing techniques~
Mindfully Get Moving

- **Make appointments.** Schedule brief social encounters for the near future, like a quick lunch or a coffee break. Avoid signing up for something that requires a lot of time. Just knowing that you will connect with someone later in the week gives you lots of time to prepare for it mentally, and it's something to look forward to. Don't cancel! It's likely that once you get there, you'll be happy you went.

- **Smile!** People are much more likely to interact with you when they see you smiling at them. It makes you very approachable.

- **Say hello to acquaintances.** Make an appointment to get your hair cut. Chitchat with your regular stylist or with a new one. Go to your favorite restaurant and say hello to the waitress who always takes your order. Strike up a conversation with the bus driver. These conversations are sure to be very light and aren't likely to push your emotional buttons.

- **Go places where people naturally gather.** Sometimes being around people can help even if you don't talk to anyone. Go to the library or wander the mall. Go to the gym and talk to the person on the treadmill next to you. Take a workshop or a class. These are good places to be around people without having to be very sociable or needing to interact with them very much.

8 soothing emergency help

If you don't know where to start or you're feeling stuck, then choose one technique from each chapter of this book and do them all. This will ensure that you soothe and comfort all the different aspects of your body and your mind. Also, if one technique doesn't work on the day you do it, be sure to try it again another time. On another day or under different circumstances, the same technique may have a beneficial outcome. An example of how to use specific techniques from each chapter is provided below.

Susan had a very tense day at work. When she got home, she was tempted to eat some leftover chocolate cake and comfort herself with food and calories. Because her craving was so strong, she knew she needed a foolproof plan. So she chose techniques from each chapter that had successfully kept her from stress eating in the recent past.

To center herself, she began with a quick breathing exercise (Breath Your Way to Inner Calm, no. 3, in chapter 3). Then she spent five minutes writing in her journal (Journaling to Boost Your Mental Health Immunity, no. 11, in chapter 4). Susan then chose to do one yoga pose (Yoga 101, no. 23, in chapter 5). She put some of her favorite music on (Meditative Music, no. 38, in chapter 6). Finally, Susan e-mailed a friend (Join the Blogosphere, no. 42, in chapter 7).

~self-soothing technique for emergency help~
Inspiration Box

Ideally, this exercise uses an empty tissue box, but any kind of empty box or jar will do. You'll be making a grab bag of techniques from this book. First, get a small stack of paper. Cut the paper into squares. On each square, write the name of one technique. Then fold each square and place it inside the box.

When you feel the urge to eat to soothe yourself, go directly to this box. Reach in and randomly pull out one folded paper square. Open it and read it. Trust the box. Commit to trying whatever technique you draw from the box. If that doesn't work, commit to drawing another square and trying that technique. If that doesn't work, commit to drawing yet another square. Practice that technique. The odds are very good that by the time you've finished doing three techniques, your urge to eat will have passed.

Important tip: Do the preparation for this technique before you are in need of using it. Have the box ready to go in times of need.

~self-soothing technique for emergency help~
Create Your Own Comfort Kit

Create a comfort kit that you can turn to when you need immediate help. Look back through this book and gather together the items you will need to complete some of the techniques. Fill a box with various items that provide soothing comfort; for example, your journal, a bottle of lotion, warm socks, a tea bag, a comfy sweater, and other items that you know will help to soothe you.

Ready, Set, Soothe

New ways to nurture yourself without food can be life changing. They can liberate you from the powerful grip of emotional eating. Before reading this book you may have continually gone to the fridge when you didn't know what else to do to heal your heavy heart. But the fridge is just a big, cold box filled with food.

It's a lousy long-term support system. Eating for comfort is like putting a Band-Aid over a gaping wound.

Finding new ways to calm down while the problem works itself out is what you need instead of food. You can use a variety of mental, physical, meditative, distracting, and social support techniques to help you through the rough moments. It may take time and practice. Be patient and persistent and you will change. You will find ways to soothe and calm yourself that do not involve eating undesirable calories. So the next time you feel strung out from a too hectic day, forget about reaching for a piece of cake. Instead, reach for this book, flip through it, and pick a soothing technique to help you feel better fast. Instead, reach for this book, flip through it, and pick a soothing technique to help you nurture and comfort yourself from this moment forward.

references

Baer, R. A. 2003. Mindfulness training as a clinical intervention: A conceptual and empirical review. *Clinical Psychology: Science and Practice* 10(2): 125-143.

Bellisle, F., and A. Dalix. 2001. Cognitive restraint can be offset by distraction, leading to increased meal intake in women. *American Journal of Clinical Nutrition* 74(2): 197-200.

Benson, H. 2001. Mind-body pioneer: The connection between your mind and body is stronger than you may think. *Psychology Today* 34(3): 56-59.

Boudette, R. 2006. Yoga in the treatment of disordered eating and body image disturbance: How can the practice of yoga be helpful in recovery from an eating disorder? *Eating Disorders* 14(2): 167-170.

Brown, K. W., R. M. Ryan, and J. D. Creswell. 2007. Mindfulness: Theoretical foundations and evidence for its salutary effects. *Psychological Inquiry* 18(4): 211-237.

Bushman, B. 2002. Does venting anger feed or extinguish the flame? Catharsis, rumination, distraction, anger, and aggressive responding. *Personality and Social Psychology Bulletin* 28(6): 724-731.

Cox N. H., R. K. Bernstein, and P. L. Hooper. 2000. Hot-tub therapy for type 2 diabetes mellitus. *New England Journal of Medicine* 342(3): 218-219.

Crum, A. J., and E. J. Langer. 2007. Mind-set matters: Exercise as a placebo. *Psychological Science* 18(2): 165-171.

Dallman, M. F., N. Pecoraro, S. F. Akana, S. E. La Fleur, F. Gomez, H. Houshyar, et al. 2003. Chronic stress and obesity: A new view of "comfort food." *Proceedings of the National Academy of Sciences* 100(20): 11696-11701.

Daubenmier, J. 2005. The relationship of yoga, body awareness, and body responsiveness to self-objectification and disordered eating. *Psychology of Women Quarterly* 29(2): 207-219.

Davidson, R. J., J. Kabat-Zinn, J. Schumacher, M. Rosenkranz, D. Muller, S. F. Santorelli, et al. 2003. Alterations in brain and immune function produced by mindfulness meditation. *Psychosomatic Medicine* 65(4): 564-570.

Epton, T., and P. R. Harris. 2008. Self-affirmation promotes health behavior change. *Health Psychology* 27(6): 746-752.

Esplen M. J., P. E Garfinkel, M. Olmsted, R. M. Gallop, and S. Kennedy. 1998. A randomized controlled trial of guided imagery in bulimia nervosa. *Psychological Medicine* 28(6): 1347-1357.

Freeman, L. M. Y., and K. M. Gil. 2004. Daily stress, coping, and dietary restraint in binge eating. *International Journal of Eating Disorders* 36(2): 204-212.

Golden, R. N., B. N. Gaynes, R. D. Ekstrom, R. M. Hamer, F. M. Jacobsen, T. Suppes, et al. 2005. The efficacy of light therapy in the treatment of mood disorders: A review and meta-analysis of the evidence. *American Journal of Psychiatry* 162(4): 656-662.

Heatherton, T. F., and R. F. Baumeister. 1991. Binge eating as an escape from self-awareness. *Psychological Bulletin* 110(1): 86-108.

Hutcherson, C. A., E. M. Seppala, and J. J. Gross. 2008. Loving-kindness meditation increases social connectedness. *Emotion* 8(5): 720-724.

Jones, K. E., R. K. Johnson, and J. R. Harvey-Berino. 2008. Is losing sleep making us obese? *Nutrition Bulletin* 33(4): 272-278.

Keeling, M. L., and M. Bermudez. 2006. Externalizing problems through art and writing: Experience of process and helpfulness. *Journal of Marital and Family Therapy.* 32(4): 405-419.

Labbé, E., N. Schmidt, J. Babin, and M. Pharr. 2007. Coping with stress: The effectiveness of different types of music. *Applied Psychophysiology and Biofeedback* 32(3-4): 163-168.

Lilienfeld, S. O., and H. Arkowitz. 2008. Can animals aid therapy? *Scientific American Mind* 19(3): 78-79.

Macht, M. 2008. How emotions affect eating: A five-way model. *Appetite* 50(1): 1-11.

Marshall, N. S., N. Glozier, and R. R. Grunstein. 2008. Is sleep duration related to obesity? A critical review of the epidemiological evidence. *Sleep Medicine Reviews* 12(4): 289-298.

Moss, M. S., L. Hewitt, L. Moss, and K. Wesnes. 2008. Modulation of cognitive performance and mood by aroma of peppermint and ylang-ylang. *International Journal of Neuroscience* 118(1): 59-77.

Parker, G., I. Parker, and H. Brotchie. 2006. Mood state effects of chocolate. *Journal of Affective Disorders* 92(2-3): 149-159.

Polivy, J., and P. Herman. 2005. Mental health and eating behaviours: A bidirectional relationship. *Canadian Journal of Mental Health* 96(S3): 43-46.

Proulx, K. 2008. Experiences of women with bulimia nervosa in a mindfulness-based eating disorder treatment group. *Eating Disorders* 16(1): 52-72.

Setter, F., and S. Kupper. 2002. Autogenic training: A meta-analysis of clinical outcome studies. *Applied Psychophysiological Biofeedback* 27(1): 45-98.

Shapiro, S. L., D. Oman, C. E. Thoresen, T. G. Plante, and T. Flinders. 2008. Cultivating mindfulness: Effects on well-being. *Journal of Clinical Psychology* 64(7): 840-862.

Spoor, S. T. P., M. H. J. Bekker, T. Van Strien, and G. L. van Heck. 2007. Relations between negative affect, coping, and emotional eating. *Appetite* 48(3): 368-376.

Steptoe, A., E. L. Gibson, R. Vuononvirta, E. D. Williams, M. Hamer, J. A. Rycroft, et al. 2006. The effects of tea on psychophysiological stress responsivity and post-stress recovery: A randomised double-blind trial. *Psychopharmacology* 190(1): 81-89.

Suomi, S. J., F. C. P. van der Horst, and R. van der Veer. 2008. Rigorous experiments on monkey love: An account of Harry F. Harlow's role in the history of attachment theory. *Integrative Psychological and Behavioral Science* 42(4): 354-369.

Thorson, J. A., F. C. Powell, I. Sarmany-Schuller, and W. P. Hampes. 1997. Psychiatric health and sense of humor. *Journal of Clinical Psychology* 53(6): 605-619.

Tugade, M. M., B. L. Fredrickson, and L. F. Barrett. 2004. Psychological resilience and positive emotional granularity: Examining the benefits of positive emotions on coping and health. *Journal of Personality* 72(6): 1161–1190.

Wansink, B., M. M. Cheney, and N. Chan. 2003. Exploring comfort food preferences across age and gender. *Physiology and Behavior* 79(4-5): 739-747.

Wardle, J., S. Sanderson, C. A. Guthrie, L. Rapoport, and R. Plomin. 2002. Parental feeding style and the intergenerational transmission of obesity risk. *Obesity Research* 10(6): 453-462.

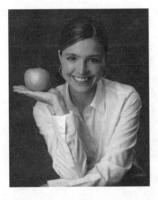

Susan Albers, Psy.D., is a licensed clinical psychologist at the Cleveland Clinic Hospital, where she specializes in eating issues, weight loss, body image concerns, and mindfulness. She graduated from the University of Denver, completed an internship at the University of Notre Dame, and was a post-doctoral fellow at Stanford University. Albers is author of Eating Mindfully, Mindful Eating 101, and Eat, Drink, and Be Mindful. She is an America Online diet and fitness coach. Albers' work has been quoted in O, The Oprah Magazine, Family Circle, Self, and the Wall Street Journal, and she conducts mindful eating workshops internationally. Visit Albers online at www.sootheyourselfwithoutfood.com.

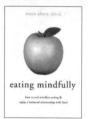
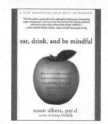
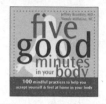
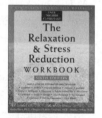
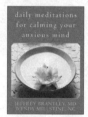